Medical Rotations: Time to Succeed

Get the Most Out of Your Training

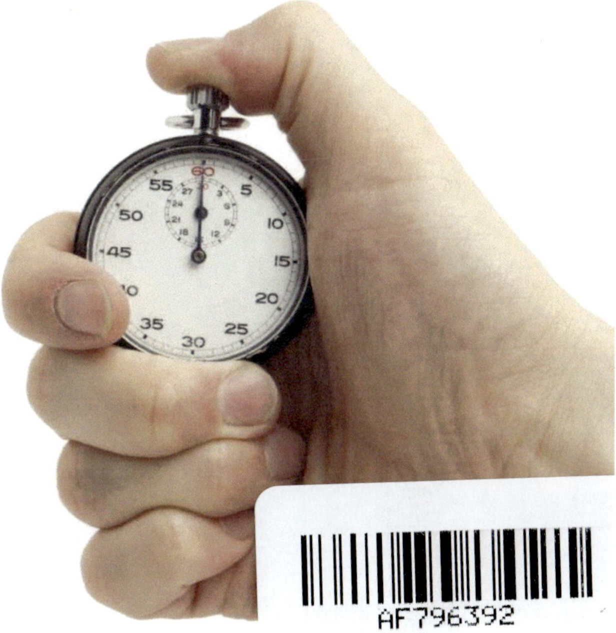

Aaron P. Shaw MS, MSBS, PA-C

Medical Rotations: Time to Succeed – Get The Most Out of Your Training
Published by Aaron P. Shaw
docashaw@gmail.com
Copy edited by Teresa M. Green

ISBN - 10: 0-692-83661-6
ISBN - 13: 978-0-692-83661-3

Printed in USA

I would like to dedicate this book to my wonderful wife, Dr. Valerie VanRavenswaay DO, MPH and our new son Jakx Shaw. You two have brought more love into my life than I have ever thought possible.

I also want to thank my family for their continued support, inspiration and love through the years. I also want to thank my brother, Jonathan Shaw PA-C, who endured PA school with me and helped me study, encouraged me and challenged me to bring my best game to medicine.

Disclaimer

This book is not intended as a substitute for the medical advice of physicians. The reader should regularly consult a physician in matters relating to his/her health and particularly with respect to any symptoms that may require diagnosis or medical attention. This book should only be used to prepare for examinations and should not be used in the practice of medicine as this material may not accurately reflect and often contradicts current medical practice.

Introduction Statement

We all know that Medical School and Physician Assistant School is very challenging. We also know that an incredible volume of information and resources are readily available on the Internet and in books at our university book stores and libraries. As I progressed through clinical rotations, I found that many books were organized based on organ systems, which made it rather frustrating and inconvenient for studying while on a time consuming medical rotation. Thus, the inspiration for this book.

I took notes on all of my medical rotations of common diseases, conditions, syndromes, and problems that I encountered, as well as the major topics that were covered on clinical rotations and that were commonly addressed on practice exams specific to these rotations. The chapters are organized by clinical rotation, and contain the topics that you will most likely encounter during that particular rotation.

This book is meant to be a review for PA and Medical students who are rotating on clinical rotations and taking shelf exams. I hope that this organization will make studying for rotations much easier and result in higher yield study sessions.

Table of Contents

Chapter One

Lab Values

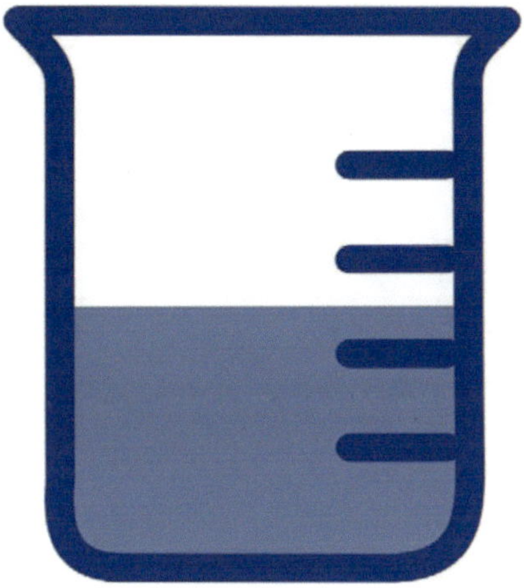

Electrolyte Panel

Ammonia	15-50 µmol/L
Ceruloplasmin	15-60 mg/dL
Chloride	95-105 mmol/L
Copper	70-150 µg/dL
Creatinine	0.8-1.3 mg/dL
Blood urea nitrogen	8-21 mg/dL
Ferritin	12-300 ng/mL (men)
	12-150 ng/mL (women)
Glucose	65-110 mg/dL
Inorganic phosphorous	1-1.5 mmol/L
Ionized calcium	1.03-1.23 mmol/L
Magnesium	1.5-2 mEq/L
Phosphate	0.8-1.5 mmol/L
Potassium	3.5-5 mmol/L
Pyruvate	300-900 µg/dL
Sodium	135-145 mmol/L
Total calcium	2-2.6 mmol/L
Total iron-binding capacity	45-85 µmol/L
Total serum iron	65-180 µg/dL (men)
	30-170 µg/dL (women)
Transferrin	200-350 mg/dL
Urea	1.2-3 mmol/L
Uric acid	0.18-0.48 mmol/L
Zinc	70-100 µmol/L

Hematology

Hemoglobin	13-17 g/dL (men)
	12-15 g/dL (women)
Hematocrit	40%-52% (men)
	36%-47% (women)
Glycosylated hemoglobin	4%-6%
Mean corpuscular volume (MCV)	80-100 fL
Red blood cell distribution width (RDW)	11.5%-14.5%
Mean corpuscular hemoglobin (MCH)	0.4-0.5 fmol/cell
Mean corpuscular hemoglobin concentration (MCHC)	30-35 g/dL
Reticulocytes	0.5%-1.5%
White blood cells (WBC)	4-10 x 10^9/L
Neutrophils	2-8 x 10^9/L
Bands	< 1 x 10^9/L
Lymphocytes	1-4 x 10^9/L
Monocytes	0.2-0.8 x 10^9/L
Eosinophils	< 0.5 x 10^9/L
Platelets	150-400 x 10^9/L
Prothrombin time	11-14 sec
International normalized ratio (INR)	0.9-1.2
Activated partial thromboplastin time (aPTT)	20-40 sec
Fibrinogen	1.8-4 g/L
Bleeding time	2-9 min

Lipid Panel

Triglycerides	50-150 mg/dL
Total cholesterol	3-5.5 mmol/L
High-density lipoprotein (HDL)	40-80 mg/dL
Low-density lipoprotein (LDL)	85-125 mg/dL

Acid Base (ABG)

pH	7.35-7.45
Base excess	(-3)-(+3)
H+	36-44 nmol/L
Partial pressure of oxygen (pO2)	75-100 mm Hg
Oxygen saturation	96%-100%
Partial pressure of carbon dioxide (pCO2)	35-45 mm Hg
Bicarbonate (HCO3)	18-22 mmol/L

Cardiac Panel

Creatine kinase	25-200 U/L
Creatine kinase MB (CKMB)	0-4 ng/mL
Troponin	0-0.4 ng/mL

Gatrointestinal Function

Albumin	35-50 g/L
Alkaline phosphatase	50-100 U/L
Alanine aminotransferase (ALT)	5-30 U/L
Amylase	30-125 U/L
Aspartate aminotransferase (AST)	5-30 U/L
Direct bilirubin	0-6 µmol/L
Gamma glutamyl transferase	6-50 U/L
Lipase	10-150 U/L
Total bilirubin	2-20 µmol/L
Total protein	60-80 g/L

Hormones

17 hydroxyprogesterone (female, follicular)	0.2-1 mg/L
Adrenocorticotropic hormone (ACTH)	4.5-20 pmol/L
Estradiol	1.5-5 ng/dL (male) 2-14 ng/dL (female, follicular) 2-16 ng/dL (female, luteal) < 3.5 ng/dL (postmenopausal)
Free T3	0.2-0.5 ng/dL
Free T4	10-20 pmol/L
Follicle-stimulating hormone (FSH)	1-10 IU/L (male) 1-10 IU/L (female follicular/luteal) 5-25 IU/L (female, ovulation) 30-110 IU/L (postmenopause)

Hormones continued

Growth hormone (fasting)	0-5 ng/mL
Progesterone	70-280 (ovulation), ng/dL
Prolactin	< 14 ng/mL
Testosterone (male)	10-25 nmol/L
Thyroxine-binding globulin	12-30 mg/L
Thyroid-stimulating hormone (TSH)	0.5-5 mIU/L
Total T4	4.9-11.7 mg/dL
Total T3	0.7-1.5 ng/dL
Free T3	0.6-1.6 ng/mL

Vitamins

Folate (serum)	7-36 nmol/L
Vitamin A	30-65 μg/dL
Vitamin B12	130-700 ng/L
Vitamin C	0.4-1.5 mg/dL
Vitamin D	5-75 ng/mL

Tumor Markers

Alpha-fetoprotein	0-44 ng/mL
Beta human chorionic gonadotropin (HCG)	< 5 IU/I
CA19.9	< 40 U/mL
Carcinoembryonic antigen (CEA)	< 4 ug/L
Prostatic acid phosphatase (PAP)	0-3 U/dL
Prostate-specific antigen (PSA)	< 4 ug/L

Miscellaneous

Alpha 1-antitrypsin	20-50 µmol/L
Angiotensin-converting enzyme	23-57 U/L
C-reactive protein	< 5 mg/L
D-dimer	< 500 ng/mL
Erythrocyte sedimentation rate (ESR)	Less than age/2 mm/hour
Lactate dehydrogenase (LDH)	50-150 U/L
Lead	< 40 µg/dL
Rheumatoid factor	< 25 IU/ml

Chapter Two

History and Physical Format (H & P)

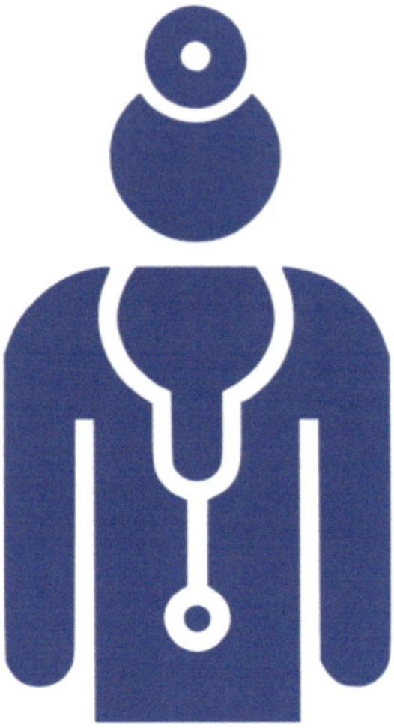

History and Physical Format (H&P)

Name, Address and Telephone #:
DOB:
Informant:
Referring provider:

CC (chief complaint)

- List of symptoms & duration
- Reason for seeking care

HPI (history of present illness) - PQRST

- **P**rovocative/palliative – precipitating/relieving
- **Q**uality/quantity – character
- **R**egion – location/radiation
- **S**everity – constant/intermittent
- **T**iming – onset/frequency/duration

PMH (Past Medical/Surgical History)

General health, weight loss, hepatitis, rheumatic fever, mono, flu, arthritis, cancer, gout, asthma/COPD, pneumonia, thyroid dx, blood dyscrasias, ASCVD, HTN, UTIs, DM, seizures, operations, injuries, PUD/GERD, hospitalizations and psychiatric history.

(**AHISTORY ++**) – Helps to remember the order

Allergies (*Side effect of medication vs. Actual hypersensitivity reaction*)

Hospitalizations (*Length of stay, any time in ICU?*)

Immunizations

Surgeries (*Minor and Major*)

Trauma (*Physical and Psychological*)

Oral medications (*Rx and OTC*)

Reproductive history (*Birth trauma, # of children, abortions, C-sections*)

Youth Illnesses

+: Screenings (*Pap smear / Colonoscopies*)

+: Vaccinations (*UTD*)

SH (Social History)

Birthplace, residence, education, occupation, marital status, ETOH, smoking, drugs, sexual activity – (*Ask, Men, Women or Both*)

CAGE Review (*Alcoholics*)

- Ever Feel Need to ***C****UT DOWN*
- Ever Felt ***A****NNOYED* by criticism of drinking
- Ever Had ***G****UILTY* Feelings
- Ever Taken Morning ***E****YE OPENER*

FH (Family History)

Age & cause of death of relatives' family diseases (*CAD, CA, DM, psych*)

SUBJECTIVE (Review of Systems)

Skin, hair, and nails: Lesions, rashes, pruritus, changes in moles; change in distribution

Lymph nodes: Enlargement, pain

Bones, joints, muscles: Fractures, pain, stiffness, weakness, atrophy

Blood: Anemia, bruising

Head: H/A, trauma, vertigo, syncope, seizures, memory

Eyes: Visual loss, diplopia, trauma, inflammation, glasses

Ears: Deafness, tinnitus, discharge, pain

Nose: Discharge, obstruction, epistaxis

Mouth: Sores, gingival bleeding, teeth, abnormal taste, jaw pain

Throat: ST, hoarseness, voice changes, URI

Neck: Swelling/stiffness, adenopathy, goiter,

Breasts: Lumps, pain, nipple discharge, last mammogram

Endocrine: Polyphagia/dipsia/uria, decreased energy/fatigue

Respiratory: Dyspnea, orthopnea, wheezing, cough, sputum, hemoptysis, pain, pleurisy, night sweats, TB, #pillows, pneumonia, asthma

CV (Cardiovascular): CP, palpitations, claudication, peripheral edema, ascites, cold feet, phlebitis, and cyanosis

GI: Appetite/ Weight change, dysphagia, N/V, hematemesis, BRBPR, melena, abdominal pain/colic, icterus, diarrhea, constipation, change in bowels, tenesmus, hemorrhoids, rectal pain, hernia

GU: Polyuria, oliguria, dysuria/straining, hematuria, pyuria, incontinence, nocturia, pain passage of stones, UTI, pyelonephritis & STD history

MS: Arthralgia, arthritis, myalgia, joint stiffness/swelling/ heat/pain, podagra/gout

Nerves: Smell, chewing, visual, facial weakness, hearing, balance, speech & swallowing, taste,

Motor: Weakness, paralysis, atrophy, seizures, incoordination

Sensory: Pain, paresthesia, and anesthesia

Autonomic: Incontinence, sweating, erythema, cyanosis, pallor, temp sensitivity

Mental status: Relations w/family, mood, hallucinations, delusions, depression, somnolence, insomnia

OBJECTIVE (Physical exam)

Vital signs & **general appearanc**e: Age, sex, well developed/nourished, appears stated age, NAD

Head: Normocephalic, no masses /lesions, cicatrices, malar flushing

Eyes: Visual fields intact, PERRLA, conjunctiva clear, sclera white, anicteric, (1-2 beat nystagmus on lateral gaze.) EOMI, no ptosis; fundi: red reflex present. Discs flat w/sharp margins, vessels present w/o crossing defects, retinal hemorrhages

Ears: TM's non-injected (erythematous, bulging), good light reflex, no protrusion or retraction; Weber midline, Rinne ac>bc, Whisper test 3:3

Nose: Nares patent, no deformity, septal deviation or perforation

Throat: Pharynx non-injected, palate rises symmetrically, gag present,

Mouth: Buccal mucosa, moist and intact, tonsils present, dentition intact, caries, tongue midline w/o fasciculations

Neck, axilla & breasts: No LAD (lymphadenopathy), masses, or thyromegaly/ focal lump, carotid pulses 2+, no bruits, supple full ROM trachea midline, breasts symmetric, no retraction, lesions, masses or tenderness

Back, thorax & lungs: Chest expansion symmetric, CTA (clear to auscultation), no adventitious sounds (rales, crackles, wheezes)

CV (cardiovascular): RRR no m/r/g (systolic ejection murmur, rubs, gallops)

Abdomen: Soft non-tender w/o masses, tympani to percussion in all 4 quads, BS present (hyper/hypoactive, absent); no HSM (hepatosplenomegaly), no bruits

Extremities: Extremity size symmetric w/o swelling/atrophy, temp warm. All pulses present, 2+, no LAD

Skin: Pink-tan color, good turgor w/o lesions, redness, cyanosis, edema or cicatrices;

Nails: No clubbing or deformities w/good capillary refill

Musculoskeletal: Gait normal, able to tandem walk, no Rhomberg's sign; joints and muscles symmetric, no swelling, masses, deformity or tenderness to palpation; no heat or swelling of joints; full ROM; muscle strength 5/5- flexion against resistance & w/o tenderness

Muscle Grading:

D (deltoid)

T (triceps)

B (biceps)

WF (wrist flexion)

WE (wrist extension)

Quad (quadriceps)

PF (plantar flexion)

DF (dorsiflexion)

Scoring 0 – 5 out of 5 according to the following scale:

- 5 Normal
- 4 Good
- 3 Fair
- 2 Poor
- 1 Trace

Range of Motion Grading:	
Complete ROM against gravity with full resistance:	5
Complete ROM against gravity with some resist:	4
Complete ROM against gravity:	3
Complete ROM with gravity eliminated:	2
Evidence of slight contractility:	1
No joint motion:	0

Genitalia/ Rectum: No lesions, inflammation or discharge from penis, rectum: no fissure, hemorrhoids, fistula or lesions in perianal area; sphincter tone good; prostate not enlarged, no masses, nodules or tenderness. Stool brown, guaiac neg.

Pelvic: No vaginal/cervical lesions, uterus size & position; no adnexal tenderness

Nervous: (LOC, DTR's, MMS) - CN II-XII grossly intact, alert oriented, cooperative

Sensory: Pinprick, light touch & vibration intact; proprioception tested (*unable to differentiate sharp/dull mid-calf*)

Motor: No atrophy, weakness, tremors or clonus; RAM (rapid, alt. movement) finger-to-nose/heel-to-shin intact; Rhomberg negative

DTR's: All 2+; Babinski absent toes upgoing, downgoing or equivocal (inconclusive); plantar response in extensor on (L); Naming & repetition intact; memory 3:3; Pronator drift - (R)>(L); gaze preference; neglect; extinguishing sensory (light touch to each extremity, then to both simultaneously): extinguishes (L or R) side to direct sensation/ stimulation. No evidence of contractility

Reflexes

Biceps (*C5, C6*)

Triceps (*C6, C7, C8*)

Brachioradialis (*C5, C6*)

Patellar (*L2, L3, L4*)

Achilles' (*S1, S2*)

Plantar/Babinski (*L4, L5, S1, S2*)

Reflex Grading Scale	
4+:	Very brisk/hyperactive: Clonus
3+:	More brisk than average
2+:	Average/normal
1+:	Low normal/diminished
0:	No response or equivocal

Cranial Nerve Evaluation - Specific Tests

CN I (*Olfactory*): Smell mint leaves/tobacco

CN II (*Optic*): Visual acuity & Funduscopic

CN III (*Occulomotor*): Pupillary reaction

CN IV (*Trochlear*): Pupillary reaction

CN V (*Trigeminal*): Clench teeth, open jaw, lip/chin test for light touch

CN VI (*Abducens*): EOM

CN VII (*Facial*): Raise eyebrow/frown/show teeth/smile/puff cheek

CN VIII (*Acoustic*): Whisper test; Weber/Rinne tests

CN IX (*Glossopharyngeal*): Hoarseness, tongue movement

CN X (*Vagus*): Saying "ah," & note palate and uvula move upward

CN XI (*Spinal Accessory*): Shrug shoulders

CN XII (*Hypoglossal*): Inspect tongue for atrophy/fasciculation's

Chapter Three

Internal Medicine

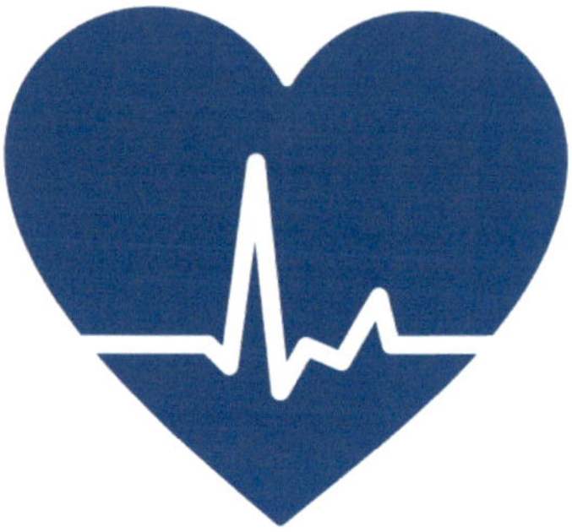

JNC Criteria for HTN w/DM

Normal:	< 120/80
Pre-HTN:	120-139/80-89
HTN 1:	140-159/90-99
HTN 2:	≥ 160/100
DM:	**< 130/80 ...often requires 2 medications to reach goal**

Post Pericardiotomy Syndrome (Dressler's Syndrome)

Definition

- Also called post myocardial infarction syndrome. This is a secondary form of pericarditis that occurs in the setting of injury to the heart or pericardium. Occurs 4-6 weeks after MI & resolves in few days.

Clinical Presentation

- Patient generally has undergone surgery that involves opening the pericardium, stab wounds, and blunt trauma to the chest, coronary artery stent placement or pacemaker implantation. This MC occurs 1-6 weeks after surgery but can happen years after surgery.
- This condition usually presents with pleuritic pain, friction rubs, pleural effusions, pneumonitis, and abnormal ECG.

Triad of features

- Fever
- Pleuritic Pain
- Pericardial Effusion/ Pericardial Friction Rub

Generally will have an elevated ESR, CRP and anti- heart antibodies

Treatment

- Typically treated with colchicine & corticosteroids or prednisone for 1 week and tapered for 4 weeks, in some resistant cases

Wernicke's Encephalopathy

Definition

- Thiamine (*vitamin B-1) deficiency* is a serious neurologic disorder. It may develop in starvation, hyperemesis gravidarum, bariatric surgery, & HIV.

Clinical Presentation

Classic Triad: 90% of patients

- Encephalopathy
- Ataxic gait
- A variant of Occulomotor dysfunction

Most of those who survive suffer from:

- Irreversible retrograde amnesia (inability to recall information)
- Anterograde amnesia (inability to assimilate new information)

Korsakoff amnestic syndrome is a late neuropsychiatric manifestation of Wernicke encephalopathy w/memory loss & confabulation related to *ETOH intake*

Treatment

- Thymine until the patient has resumed a regular diet. Administer *daily oral thiamine* (100 mg) on a long-term, outpatient basis.
- Treat with empiric *parenteral magnesium sulfate* so that the patient will be able to absorb the thiamine more effectively. The patient is most likely deficient in Mg anyways.

Overriding Clavicle/ AC Separation

Definition

- The Acromion-Clavicular joint is located at the top of the shoulder where the acromion process and the clavicles meet to form a joint. The ligaments holding this joint together may tear and the joint will separate.

Type I	Involve minimal disruption of the acromioclavicular joint and are intrinsically stable.
Type II	The acromioclavicular ligament is completely torn.
Type III	Acromioclavicular injuries have complete tearing of both the coracoclavicular and acromioclavicular ligaments
Type IV	The deltotrapezial fascia is disrupted in addition to complete tears of the acromioclavicular and coracoclavicular ligaments.

Clinical Presentation

Overriding Clavicle

- These *high-energy fractures are not common in most sports* & are no longer considered a minor one and displaced fractures that heal crooked will, in many cases, cause permanent problems such as pain, weakness, and deformity. Severe displacement, characterized by overriding of the fragments, fracture fragments threatening to pierce the skin, multiple fractures in the extremity, associated nerve injury, multiple rib fractures, or fractures close to the shoulder end of the clavicle.

AC Separation

- Problems often occur to this joint as a result of a *fall or impact to the outside part of the shoulder*. Often called an AC separation, these injuries are *seen most often in contact sports* and in biking and skiing falls. When an AC separation occurs, patients will complain of pain and the presence of a bump on the top of the shoulder.

Treatment

- Type I and II injuries are generally treated non-operatively in the acute setting.
- Types IV-VI injuries generally require surgical repair.

Chronic Obstructive Pulmonary Disease

Definition

- The presence of airflow limitation, measured by forced expiratory volume in 1 second (FEV_1) Chronic inflammation present in the lungs of patients with COPD leads to narrowing of small airways, destruction of parenchymal tissues, and other structural changes.

- Must have the presence of a chronic productive cough for 3 months during each of 2 consecutive years (other causes of cough being excluded).

Clinical Presentation

- Classically patients will present with air trapping, hyperinflation, and mucus hyper secretion. "*Blue Bloaters*". Patients will have increased chest diameter. May also have peripheral edema and cyanosis (Clubbing).

  Cough is worst in the morning with productive colorless sputum.

  Acute chest illness

  Breathlessness, the most significant symptom, but usually does not occur until the sixth decade of life.

  Wheezing may occur in some patients, particularly during exertion and exacerbations.

  Spirometry is the *"gold standard"* for diagnosing and monitoring the progression of COPD.

Treatment

- STOP Smoking!!

Stage I (mild obstruction)	Decrease risk factors (influenza vaccine)
Stage II (moderate obstruction)	Short + long acting bronchodilators
Stage III (severe obstruction)	Short +Long acting bronchodilators and add inhaled glucocorticoids
Stage IV (very severe obstruction or moderate obstruction with evidence of chronic respiratory failure)	Short +Long acting bronchodilators + inhaled glucocorticoids + long term Oxygen therapy and consider lung transplant

DeQuervain's Tenosynovitis

Definition

- This is a *tenosynovitis of the sheath or tunnel* that surrounds two tendons that control movement of the thumb. Idiopathic. AKA: gamer's thumb, washerwoman's sprain, or radial styloid tenosynovitis

Clinical Presentation

- Symptoms are pain, tenderness, and swelling over the thumb side of the wrist, and difficulty gripping

Physical Exam

- *Finkelstein's test* is used to diagnose de Quervain syndrome in people who have wrist pain. To perform the test, the examining physician grasps the thumb and the hand is ulnar deviated sharply. If sharp pain occurs along the distal radius de Quervain's syndrome is likely.

Treatment

- *Corticosteroid injection* is the first line of treatment. Surgery should be reserved for unsuccessful injections.

Nephrotic Syndrome

Definition

- Is a nonspecific disorder in which the kidneys are damaged, causing them to leak large amounts of protein from the blood into the urine & subsequently hypoalbuminemia, because some of the protein albumin has gone from the blood to the urine

Clinical Presentation

Patients present with:

- Proteinuria (>3.5g/day)
- Hypoalbuminemia
- Hyperlipidemia
- Edema (anasarca or dropsy) that begins in the face
- Lipiduria can also occur. No hematuria

The gold standard in diagnosis of Nephrotic syndrome is 24-hour urine protein measurement *with 2 g of protein per gram of urine creatinine*

Primary Causes

- Minimal-change nephropathy
- Focal glomerulosclerosis
- Membranous nephropathy
- Hereditary nephropathies

Treatment

Treatment is dependent on the cause.

- *Corticosteroids* (prednisone), cyclophosphamide, and cyclosporine are used to induce remission in Nephrotic syndrome
- *Diuretics* are used to reduce edema
- *Angiotensin-converting enzyme (ACE)* inhibitors and angiotensin II receptor blockers are administered to reduce proteinuria

Nephritic Syndrome

Definition

- This is inflammation of the kidneys. A collection of signs associated with disorders affecting specifically glomerular disorders. RBCs pass through the pores, causing hematuria.

Clinical Presentation

Patients have complaints of hematuria or oliguria. Nephritic syndrome is characterized by:

- *Hematuria* (blood in the urine)
- *Proteinuria* - small amounts, usually trivial (<3.5 g/day)
- *Hypertension (mild), & uremia* - due to retention of waste products

This is a clinical syndrome w/o a specific diagnosis.

Treatment

Treatment is dependent on the cause.

- *Corticosteroids* (prednisone), cyclophosphamide, and cyclosporine are used to induce remission in Nephrotic syndrome
- *Diuretics* are used to reduce edema
- *Angiotensin-converting enzyme (ACE)* inhibitors and angiotensin II receptor blockers are administered to reduce proteinuria

Auer Rods

Definition

- These are elongated structures seen in malignant cells of the neutrophil lineage. These are mostly seen in myeloblasts, which are found only in acute myeloid leukemias (AML), either myeloblastic or monoblastic. So if you see blasts with Auer rods, you know it is some type of acute myeloid leukemia.

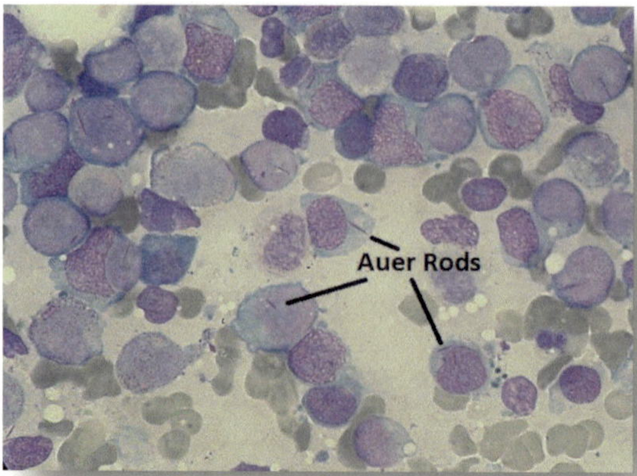

Figure 1: By Paulo Henrique Orlandi Mourao - Own work, CC BY-SA 3.0

Chronic Myelogenous Leukemia

Definition

- This is a myeloproliferative disorder characterized by increased proliferation of the granulocytic cell line without the loss of their capacity to differentiate. CML represents 20 % of all Adult Leukemia.

Clinical Presentations

- Patients present with fatigue, weight loss, excessive sweating, low-grade fever, hepatomegaly, LUQ pain d/t spleen infarction. They can also have anemia, bleeding and bone pain in the blast phase.

Labs

- Total WBC count 20,000-60,000 cells/μL, with mildly increased basophils and eosinophils
- Philadelphia (Ph) chromosome in bone marrow cells
- *BCR/ABL* mutation
- Megakaryocytes are prominent and may be increased
- Increased blasts >20% typically

Meningitis

Definition

- This is inflammation of the membranes (meninges) surrounding the brain and spinal cord. MCC is viral infection, but can be bacterial or fungal.

Clinical Presentation

- **Hallmark S/S**: 1. Headache 2. Fever 3.Stiff neck

Patients can present with photophobia, N/V, Sleepiness, Seizures and stiff neck.

- *50%* of patients with pneumococcal meningitis also *have evidence of pneumonia* on initial chest radiography.

Labs

- CT of the head before Lumbar puncture to determine risk of herniation
- Test for syphilis
- Blood cultures and blood smear

Treatment

- Viral usually resolves on its own. Bacterial must be Tx w/Antibiotic: PCN, Cefotaxime, Rosephin, & Vanco for resistant cases.

- Begin *empiric antibiotic coverage* according to age and presence of overriding physical conditions. Empiric therapy also depends on prevalence of *cephalosporin-resistant S pneumonia (DRSP)*.

Heart Murmurs

- Heart murmurs generally are heard d/t congenital abnormalities, cardiac shunts or valve abnormalities

Other causes: Rheumatic Fever, Pericarditis, Valve Calcification, or Mitral Valve Prolapse.

Treatment

- Dependent on condition: w/digoxin, anticoagulants, diuretics, ACE-I, Statins, or B-blockers. Can be crescendo, decrescendo or crescendo decrescendo.

Mitral valve prolapse: Leads to regurgitation

Mitral valve or aortic stenosis

- Stenosis can wear out your heart and can lead to heart failure
- Mitral and aortic stenosis can occur as calcium is deposited on the valves as people age

Aortic sclerosis

- Usually due to scarring, thickening, or stiffening (sclerosis) of the aortic valve, without evidence of narrowing, or stenosis
- Aortic sclerosis is usually seen in *people with atherosclerosis*, or hardening of the arteries

Mitral or aortic regurgitation

- Occurs with *mitral valve prolapse* or *aortic stenosis*
- The heart has to work harder to force blood through the damaged valve
- Leads to weaken and/or enlarge the heart and can lead to heart failure

Holosytolic Murmurs

This sound *begins immediately with S1 and continues up to S2*

1. Mitral valve regurgitation: Loudest at the left ventricular apex, usually associated with a systolic thrill, a soft S3, and a short diastolic rumbling
2. Tricuspid valve regurgitation
3. Ventricular septal defect

Diastolic Murmurs

This is *almost always indicative of heart disease*

- **Aortic Regurgitation**
  - High pitched, decrescendo, Blowing quality
  - Can signify regurgitate flow through an incompetent semilunar valve
- **Mitral Stenosis**
  - Murmur begins with "opening snap"
  - S1 accentuated, rumbling diastolic murmur in mid/late diastole, suggest stenosis of an AV valve

Systolic Murmurs

1. Aortic stenosis - Ejection type
2. Mitral regurgitation - Holosytolic
3. Mitral valve prolapse - late systole

Diastolic Murmurs

1. Aortic regurgitation - early diastole
2. Mitral stenosis - mid to late diastole

S1	Closing of the AV Valves – Mitral & Tricuspid
S2	Closing of the Semilunar Valves – Aortic & Pulmonary
S3	"*Kentucky*"
	Ventricular gallop or a proto-diastolic gallop because of its place in early diastole
	Middle-aged or older adult= S_3 is often a sign of disease, indicating increased ventricular filling due to *congestive heart failure* or severe mitral or tricuspid regurgitation
S4	"*Tennessee*" The S_4 sound occurs immediately before S_1, while the atria of the heart is vigorously contracting
	S_4 is caused by stiffening of the walls of the ventricles, which produces an abnormally turbulent flow as the atria contract to force blood into the ventricle
	Best heard as a "split S1"

Pulmonary Embolism

Definition

- Usually arise from thrombi that originate in the deep venous system of the lower extremities.
- MC get lodged in a bifurcation of two arteries or in distal pulmonary arteries

Clinical Presentation

- Unexplained shortness of breath, Pleuritic chest pain that gets worse with a deep breath, and coughing up blood. Tachycardia.

Treatment

- Patient needs a CT scan of the chest or MRA of chest if contraindicated with pacemaker
- Oral Warfarin at time of diagnosis
- LMWH after INR is within therapeutic range of 2-3 only after 5 days of warfarin therapy

Arthritis

Osteoarthritis

Definition

- A group of mechanical abnormalities involving degradation of joints, including articular cartilage and subchondral bone
- OA: MC form of arthritis, and the leading cause of chronic disability in the United States

Clinical Presentation

- Joint pain, tenderness, stiffness, locking, and sometimes an effusion.
- Caused by hereditary, developmental, metabolic, and mechanical reasons and may initiate processes leading to loss of cartilage

Treatment

- Use a combination of exercise, lifestyle modification, and analgesics.
- First line: Acetaminophen / paracetamol and NSAIDs are only recommended as add on therapy if pain relief is not sufficient
- Cortisone (Kenalog 40mg) w/ 1% Lidocaine for pain relief
- Debilitating pain: Joint replacement surgery may be used to improve the quality of life
- Hard bony enlargements: *Heberden's nodes* (distal interphalangeal joints)
- *Bouchard's nodes* (proximal interphalangeal joints)
- X-rays may confirm the diagnosis. The typical changes seen on X-ray include: joint space narrowing, subchondralsclerosis, subchondral cyst formation, and osteophytes.

Fibromyalgia

Clinical Presentation

- Chronic widespread pain and allodynia as well as tingling of the skin, prolonged muscle spasms, weakness in the limbs, nerve pain, muscle twitching, palpitations, functional bowel disturbances, and chronic sleep disturbances.

Treatment

- CBT, Antidepressants, & Pregabalin have proven to help Tx.
- NSAIDS are NOT indicated

Gout

Definition

- Recurrent attacks of acute inflammatory arthritis

Clinical Presentation

- Red, tender, hot, swollen joint. The metatarsal-phalangeal joint at the base of the big toe is the most commonly affected
- Also presents as tophi, kidney stones, or urate nephropathy

- Caused by elevated levels of uric acid in the blood. The uric acid crystallizes, and the crystals deposit in joints, tendons, and surrounding tissues. Hyperuricemia is the underlying cause ofgout.
- Renal under excretion of uric acid is the primary cause of hyperuricemia

Treatment

- NSAIDs are the first-line treatment
- Acute: Colchicine is an alternative for those unable to tolerate NSAIDs. Glucocorticoids = NSAIDs for effectiveness.
- Chronic: Allopurinol for life

Rheumatoid Arthritis

Definition

- Chronic, systemic inflammatory disorder that may affect many tissues and organs, but principally attacks (synovial) joints
- RA is a systemic autoimmune disease and nearly always affects multiple joints, most commonly small joints of the hands, feet and cervical spine, but larger joints like the shoulder and knee can also be involved

Treatment

- Disease-Modifying Anti-Rheumatic Drugs (*DMARDs*) are required to inhibit or halt the underlying immune process and prevent long-term damage

Systemic Lupus Erythematous

Definition

- Systemic Autoimmune Disease; SLE affects the heart, joints, skin, lungs, blood vessels, liver, kidneys, and nervous system.

Treatment

- There is **no cure** for SLE; however, it is treated with immunosuppression, mainly with *cyclophosphamide, corticosteroids and other immunosuppressants*. SLE is one of several diseases known as "*the great imitators*".

Diagnosis: Need (4 of 11)

- Malar Rash
- Discoid rash
- Serositis
- Oral ulcers
- Arthritis
- Photosensitivity
- Blood—hematologic disorder—hemolytic anemia, leukopenia, lymphopenia, or thrombocytopenia
- Renal disorder
- Antinuclear antibody test positive
- Immunologic disorder
- Neurologic disorder

Post-Menopausal Bleeding

Definition

- This is abnormal bleeding after cessation of menopause
- Average age of menses cessation is 51

Clinical Presentation

- Post-menopausal bleeding is *CA* until proven otherwise
- 10% - 15% of women with PMB have an endometrial carcinoma, so this should be taken seriously
- The MCC of postmenopausal bleeding is *vaginal atrophy*

Treatment

- *Always* do an endometrial biopsy

Sinus Infection

Definition

- The inflammation of the paranasal sinuses, which may be due to infection, allergy, or autoimmune issues.
- MCC= Viral
- MCC Bacterial: S. Pneumo, H. Fluenza, M. Catarrhalis
- MCC Fungal: Aspergillus

Clinical Presentation

- Allergic: *Red nasal turbinate's, eosinophilia*
- Runny nose, watery eyes, maxillary and frontal sinus tenderness, postnasal discharge, persistent cough and pharyngeal irritation, fatigue, ear pressure, fever and halitosis

Treatment

- Nasal irrigation= chronic
- Decongestant nasal sprays: However, use these medications no more than the recommended period.
- *Amoxicillin*: First line
- Fluoroquinolones or a tetracycline's, for those who have severe allergies to penicillin's, or for first line treatment failure

Beta-Blocker

BB Contraindicated

- Patients with *asthma*, especially non-selective BB d/t moa @ B1 & B2. B2 is in the lungs, B1 mostly in heart.
- Avoid in patients with a *history of cocaine* use or in cocaine-induced tachycardia.
    - Cocaine puts the body in fight or flight mode because it blocks the reuptake of NorEpi & Dopamine, increasing sympathetic drive = increased heart rate, O2 demand, & peripheral vasoconstriction.
    - Cocaine + BB leads to unopposed Alpha effect, which will cause peripheral vasoconstriction & coronary artery vasoconstriction- MI.
    - Cocaine caused cardiac vasospasm & increases O2 demand.
    - BB should not be used in *CHF* because reduces heart rate & cardiac output.

Coarctation of the Aorta

Definition

- A congenital condition: Aorta narrows in the area where the ductus arteriosus inserts.

- Classically located *distal to the origin of the left subclavian artery*.
- *Dilatation of the descending aorta immediately distal to the Coarctation*

Clinical Presentation

- MC has a ductus arteriosus, VSD and aortic stenosis.
- Congestive heart failure, severe acidosis and poor perfusion to the lower body
- Later: hypertension, headache, nosebleed, leg cramps, muscle weakness, cold feet, or neurologic changes can be noted.

Treatment

- Be conservative if *asymptomatic*
- May require *surgical resection* of the narrow aorta if there is arterial hypertension
- *Angioplasty* can be performed to dilate the narrowed artery

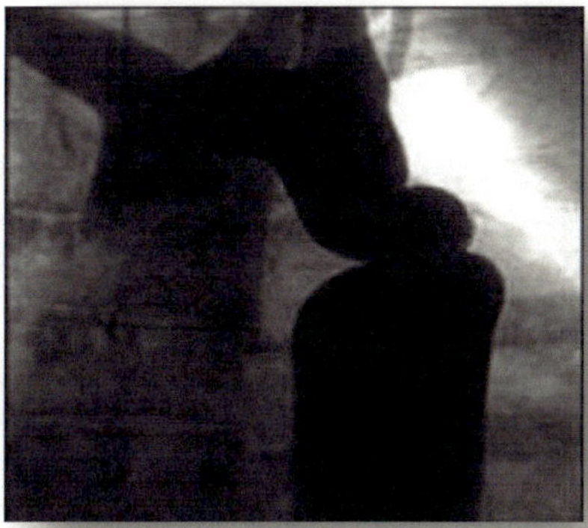

Figure 2: from Medscape, Aortic Coarctation Imaging, Nov. 24, 2015.

Cirrhosis Signs

Definition

- This is the inflammation of the liver that results in liver damage
- MC caused by alcoholism, hepatitis B, and hepatitis C, & fatty liver disease and many other possible causes. Some cases are idiopathic.

Clinical Presentation

- Jaundice due to bilirubin in the blood, fatigue, weakness and loss of appetite
- Bruising from decreased production of blood clotting factors by the diseased liver
- Edema & Ascites, Spontaneous Bacterial Peritonitis (SBP), Bleeding from Esophageal Varices, Hepatic Encephalopathy, Hepatorenal Syndrome, Hepatopulmonary Syndrome, Hypersplenism, & Liver CA.
- Increased AFP on labs= sign of liver damage

Treatment

- Depends on type of hepatitis

Anti-Depressant Side Effects

Definition

- Major depression: clinically depressed for more than 2 weeks

Clinical Presentation

- Nausea, increased appetite, weight gain, sexual side effects, fatigue, drowsiness, insomnia, dry mouth, blurred vision, constipation, dizziness, & agitation

Treatment

- Some SE resolves within a couple of weeks of starting meds, if they persist past 6 weeks, treatment needs to be re-evaluated

Cardiac Tamponade

Definition

- An accumulation of fluid in the pericardial space with reduced ventricular filling and hemodynamic compromise
- Medical emergency if acute: fast bleed
- Keep close watch if slow bleed

Clinical Presentation

- Weight loss, fatigue, anorexia, fever, elevated JVP, and chest pain

Treatment

- Initial management in hospital is by pericardiocentesis.
- Surgical pericardiectomy or pericardial window may also be done

Also all patients should receive:

1. Oxygen
2. Volume expansion with blood, plasma, dextran, or isotonic sodium chloride solution, as necessary for adequate intravascular volume
3. Bed rest with leg elevation: increase venous return
4. Inotropic drugs (Dobutamine): Increases cardiac output without increasing systemic vascular resistance

Positive-pressure mechanical ventilation should be avoided because it may decrease venous return and aggravate signs and symptoms of tamponade

Tuberculosis

Definition

- Mycobacterium tuberculosis; a small, aerobic, non-motile bacillus
- The Mantoux tuberculin skin test is often used to screen people at high risk for TB

Clinical Presentation

- Cough (lasts three or more weeks), Unintentional weight loss, Fatigue, Fever, Night sweats, Chills, Loss of appetite, Coughing up blood or sputum, Chest pain, or pain with breathing or coughing
- Most infections are *asymptomatic and latent*, but about one in ten latent infections eventually progresses to active disease which kills more than 50% of those so infected
- Classic TB: chronic cough with blood-tinged sputum, fever, night sweats, and weight loss

Treatment

Mantoux (+): **> 5mm:** HIV, immunosuppressed, organ transplant or fibrotic changes

> 10 mm: IV drug users, recent immigrants, high-risk employees, children < 4

> 15 mm: Everyone

- *Four- drug regimen*: isoniazid, rifampin, pyrazinamide, and either ethambutol or streptomycin
- After 2 months, treat for 4 months with isoniazid and rifampin

Diabetes S/S & Treatment

Type 1 Diabetes

- Frequent urination
- Unusual thirst
- Extreme hunger
- Unusual weight loss
- Extreme fatigue and Irritability

Type 2 Diabetes

- Any of the type 1 symptoms
- Frequent infections
- Blurred vision
- Cuts/bruises that are slow to heal
- Tingling/numbness in the hands/feet
- Recurring skin, gum, or bladder infections

DM can lead to diabetic neuropathy, gastroparesis, retinopathy, & CV disease in the long run.

Diagnosis

- Pre DM: A1C= 6- 6.4
- DM: A1C > 6.4

Treatment

- Lifestyle changes always first (including *diet, exercise and weight control*)
- *Metformin*: Inhibit the release of glucagon from the liver & increases insulin sensitivity
  - Promotes weight loss & lowers LDL
- *Insulin injections*, often multiple drugs both oral & SQ

Acne Vulgaris

Definition

- Common chronic skin disease involving blockage and/or inflammation of sebaceous units (hair follicles and their accompanying sebaceous gland)

Clinical Presentation

- Commonly have comedones (white heads), papules, pustules, and nodules in a sebaceous distribution (face, upper chest, back)

Treatment

- Benzoyl Peroxide or Salicylic Acid
- Benzoclyin or Duac (Benzoyl Peroxide & Clindamycin) good topical agent
- Tetracycline (Doxy or Minocyclin) is the oral antibiotic drug of choice for moderate to severe acne
- Retinoid/Retinoic Acids: Photosensitivity & peeling of the skin
- *Accutane/ ISOTRETINOIN: SE*→ Benign cerebral hypertension, TERATOGENESIS, Category X

Pyelonephritis vs. Glomerulonephritis

Pyelonephritis

Definition

- Inflammation of the upper UG tract (kidneys, renal pelvis, parenchyma and bladder)

Clinical Presentation

- FEVER, chills, Flank pain, N/V

Treatment

Long term abx: (~14+ days)

- **Uncomplicated**: *Outpatient care*: Levaquin 500 mg daily x 14 days or Cipro 500 mg, twice daily
- **Complicated:** *Inpatient care*: IV abx (IV Fluoroquinolone or Ampicillin (2g q6hrs) + gentamicin (1.5mg/kg q8hrs) then continue until afebrile 24-48 hrs

    - After discharge: Oral antibiotic x 14 days
    - Levaquin or Cipro – culture specif. F/u required! Urine culture 4-6 weeks after
    - (10-30% will need an additional 14 days of abx)

Glomerulonephritis

Definition

- Inflammation in the glomerulus; often caused by other diseases, and leads to nephritic syndrome.

Clinical Presentation

- *Azotemia* (↑ BUN in the blood), Oliguria, Hematuria, Foamy urine (from protein), Generalized edema, HTN, Blood in the vomit or stools, SOB/cough, Fever, Nosebleed, Generalized sick feeling
- *Classic= Hematuria, proteinuria (<3.5 g/day), and often HTN*

Diagnosis

- RBC casts, Decreased GFR, UA (Azotemia, oliguria, hematuria, proteinuria)
- Images: CT/Xray/US/IVP

Treatment

Anti-HTN, Corticosteroids, Plasmaphoresis and kidney transplant

Pneumonia

Definition

- Characterized by fluid in the lungs
- Can be d/t aspiration, viral, bacterial or fungal infections

Clinical Presentation

- Cough, sputum, fever, chills, left-sided pain, had a sore throat
- Often can hear egophony and lower lobe crackles and rales/ dull to percussion.
- Common killer of elderly patients

Treatment

- **Lower airways**: Bacterial > Viral, Airway consolidation, Dyspnea
    - Antibiotics = YES

Imaging

- CXR: PA and lateral reveal severe airspace opacification
- Often there is blunting of the costophrenic angles representing pleural fluid
- The cardiac silhouette may not be seen.
- Ground glass & Diffuse infiltrate common on CXR

Labs: Increased WBC w/Left shift

Viral: This has a prolonged onset, more vague presentation and is not as fast or severe as bacterial

Hospital-acquired pneumonia: 48 hrs. after hospital admission

The most common pathogens are *gram-negative bacilli* and *Staphylococcus aureus*

Tetralogy of Fallot

Definition

Congenital defect: MC cyanotic heart disease (*4 abnormalities*)

- Pulmonary Stenosis
- Overriding Aorta: aorta connects to R & L ventricles

- Ventricular Septal Defect
- Right Ventricular Hypertrophy

Clinical Presentation

- Difficulty eating
- Failure to thrive
- Dyspnea
- "Tet" spells (cyanotic skin) during feeding and crying

Treatment

- Oxygen
- Surgery if progressive (typically before age 1)

Anemia

Aplastic Anemia

- (Normocytic, Normochromic) - Suppression of multipotent myeloid stem cells leading to marrow failure and pancytopenia
- NO SPLENOMEGALY
- CBC→ (↓RBC, WBC, and platelets)
- Peripheral blood smear → decreased WBC's
- Reticulocyte count → decreased
- Bone Marrow: Hypoplastic marrow with increased fat

B12 Deficiency

- Lack of vitamin B12 (Cobalamin) d/t malabsorption (*lack of intrinsic factor – Pernicious Anemia*) or a lack in dietary intake
- Pernicious Anemia: MC
- (Macrocytic Anemia)
- ↓ B12, ↑ Fe, ↑ LDH & Bilirubin
- Shilling test→ determines etiology
    - Symptoms: *Neurologic problems*→ numbness, parastheia, weakness, ataxia
    - Angular chilitis, Pale, Glossitis, Anorexia

Folate Deficiency

- MC due to decreased intake, increased need, pregnancy, Celiac Sprue, excess alcohol
- *No Neurological Symptoms*
- Angular chilitis, Pale, Glossitis, Anorexia
- Macrocytic anemia, ↓ RBC folic acid

Iron Deficiency

- MCC of Anemia worldwide
- Chronic Blood loss, inadequate iron intake, reproduction & growth
- **Lab**: Blood Smear: Microcytic, hypochromic anemia, Erythrocytes smaller than lymphocyte nucleus
  - ↓ Serum Fe, ↓ Serum ferritin, ↑ Total iron-binding capacity (TIBC)
  - Bone marrow biopsy (*GOLD STANDARD*): Absence of iron
- **Symptoms:** Weakness, Pallor, Dizziness, Decreased exercise tolerance, Dysphagia, Pica, Glossitis, Koilonychias

Hemolytic Anemia

- IgG antibodies tag the RBC for destruction by macrophages.
- Develops slowly, Jaundice, Dark urine, Weakness, Fatigable (Normocytic anemia)
- **Blood Smear:** Spherocytes, polychromasia, nucleated RBC's, Large, Blue tinged red cells
- **Lab:** ↑ Reticulocyte Count, + Coombs test, ↓ Haptoglobin, ↑ LDH and Indirect bilirubin
- **Treatment:** Corticosteroids, Splenectomy, Cold agglutinin (avoid cold temperatures)

Hepatitis Immunizations

Schedule

- Dosing schedule is 0 (in hospital), 2 and 6 months
- Hep A vaccine recommended at age 12 months

- Combined Hep A + B vaccine for 18 years and older that will need Hep A coverage for travel or child-care workers
- Confirm immunizations with titers
- Inactivated virus is ok to give to immune-compromised patients.
- There are no studies in pregnant women- Cat C
- Positive anti-HBs with negative anti-HBc seen with immunity from immunization
- If you have surface antigen with antibodies, then you are infectious.
- Core can only be + with infection

AB	+ or -	Result
HBsAg	(-)	Immune d/t natural infection
Anti-HBc	(+)	
Anti-HBs	(+)	
HBsAg	(-)	Immune d/t HepB Vaccine
Anti-HBc	(-)	
Anti-HBs	(+)	

High risk for Hepatitis B: (recommended vaccination)

- Sexually transmitted disease treatment facilities
- HIV testing and treatment facilities
- Facilities providing drug-abuse treatment and prevention services
- Health care settings targeting services to injection drug users
- Correctional facilities
- Health care settings targeting services to men who have sex with men
- Chronic hemodialysis facilities and end-stage renal disease programs
- Institutions and nonresidential day care facilities for developmentally disabled persons
- New cases have decreased approximately 81% since 1991 when the recommendations began for immunizing all infants
- Booster doses are recommended for hemodialysis patients and other immune compromised persons

Rashes: See

http://www.webmd.com/skin-problems-and-treatments/ss/slideshow-common-adult-skin-problems

Closed Angle Glaucoma

Definition

- A rapid or sudden increase in IOP in which the iris gets pushed up against the trabecular meshwork and blocks drainage of the aqueous humor
- MC in Asians, women and elderly

Clinical Presentation

- *Medical emergency* that can lead to blindness
- Severe eye pain, headache, N/V, excessive tearing, blurred vision or **HALOS** around lights
- Normal IOP is *10-21 mmHg*. With acute closed angle glaucoma, it can reach *40-80 mmHg*

Treatment

- Acetazolamide stat dose: 500 mg IV followed by 500 mg PO
- A dose of a topical beta-blocker (Carteolol, Timolol) will also aid in lowering IOP
- If more of a decrease in IOP is needed addition of an alpha agonist may help
- A laser iridotomy is the most commonly performed surgical procedure for treatment

COPD vs. Asthma

Obstructive Diseases

COPD mainly affects the large airways and is defined as the presence of a chronic productive cough for *3 months during each of 2 consecutive years*

Asthma mainly affects the medium and small airways and has *eosinophils* associated with the pathology

- If spirometry confirms airway obstruction, the main differential diagnoses are COPD and Asthma

- Dyspnea, chronic cough and sputum production in an adult with a history of smoking or exposure to noxious particles or gases favors COPD

- A history of *childhood wheezing, atopic symptoms and diurnal variation in peak flows* (as established by monitoring at home twice daily for 2 weeks) in an adult who coughs, wheezes or is short of breath favors a diagnosis of asthma

- *An improvement in FEV1 after bronchodilator of 12%* (200ml) of exhaled air favors a diagnosis of *asthma*, but that can sometimes occur in COPD, so some experts favor an increase of *400 ml* after treatment trial to be certain of asthma as the diagnosis

- If there is uncertainty, consider a *therapeutic trial of prednisone* 30 mg daily for 2 weeks or of inhaled corticosteroids for 2-4 weeks. A marked improvement in FEV1 (> 400 ml) favors the diagnosis of asthma

- COPD in the symptomatic patient is suggested by a post-bronchodilator *FEV1 /FVC <0.7*

- *Asthma* determined by the presence of *reversibility* or (*>12% improvement*) in FEV1 and at least a 200ml increase post bronchodilator

- If fully reversible (to normal values) treat as asthma

If COPD, *grade severity*

FEV1% of predicted post-bronchodilator	
ƒ >80%	Mild
ƒ 50-80%	Moderate
ƒ 30-50%	Severe
ƒ <30%	Very Severe

Ischemic Stroke vs. Hemorrhagic Stroke

Ischemic

- More common than hemorrhagic
- Sudden loss of blood circulation to an area of the brain, resulting in a corresponding loss of neurologic function
- Caused by a thrombotic or embolic occlusion
- Sometimes preceded by a TIA
- Treat BP if *systolic blood pressure is higher than 220 mm Hg or diastolic blood pressure above 120 mm Hg*

Treatment

- If within 3 hours use rt-PA to break the blockage up.
- Carotid endardectomy or other endovascular techniques
- Use induced hypothermia for Neuroprotection

Hemorrhagic

- This is characterized by bleeding that occurs directly into the brain parenchyma
- *MCC is chronic hypertension*
- Innocence= 8-18%

Treatment

- Anticonvulsants: To prevent seizures d/t pressure on the brain
- Antihypertensive agents: To reduce BP and other risk factors of heart disease
- Osmotic diuretics: To decrease intracranial pressure in the subarachnoid space
- May also need burr holes drilled in skull or evacuation of the blood to decrease the ICP
- Avoid rt-PA (*Contraindicated*) will kill the patient

Imaging

- *CT is gold standard*, MRI may be needed if there is a trauma and the spine is involved
- Workup: Carotid duplex, EKG (looking for A-fib), brain angiography, Echo, MRA and/or CTA

Cholesterol Screening

Recommendations

- *USPSTF*: Start screening men aged *20-35 with risk factors* for CAD and women 20-45 with risk factors
- Otherwise, start screening at *35 in men or 45 in women*. Continue screening until age 65
- Screening is *every 5 years for those at low risk* of CAD, *2-4 years for those at moderate risk*, and *yearly for those at high risk*
    - (Based on Framingham risk assessment)

Type	Goals
LDL (Low Density)	<100
HDL (High Density)	<40-60>
Total Cholesterol	<200

Acute Pancreatitis

Definition

- Inflammation of the pancreas in which enzymes can be released that auto-digest the glands

Clinical Presentation

- Abdominal pain, which is characteristically dull, boring, and steady
- The pain is *sudden in onset* and gradually intensifies in severity until reaching a constant ache
- MC pain is located in the *upper abdomen*, in the *epigastric region*
- Cholelithiasis (MCC= 45%)
- ALT >150 = gallstone pancreatitis

Lab

- Lipase> 3x normal= Acute pancreatitis

Treatment

- NPO
- IV Hydration: several L bolus, then 250-500ml/hr. IV infusion
- Analgesics for pain

Other Causes

"*I GET SMASHED*" – Idiopathic, Gallstones, ETOH, Alcohol, Tumors, Scorpion stings, Microbacterial, Autoimmune (SLE & Crohn's), Surgery/Trauma, Emboli, Drugs/Toxins

Common Genetic Hematologic Disorders

VWF	MC Hereditary *Bleeding* Disorder
Factor V Leiden	Most common inherited *hypercoagulable* condition
Thalassemia	Mostly affects Mediterranean heritage
Sickle cell anemia	Mostly affects African Americans—can cause resistance to malaria

Heart Failure Causes

Definition

- Develops when the heart, via abnormal cardiac function, fails to pump blood at a rate that meets the requirements of the metabolizing tissues or is able to do so only with an elevated diastolic filling pressure
- CAD causes 2/3 of cases

- Causes= chronic HTN (diastolic dysfunction), valvular heart disease, hypertrophic cardiomyopathy, and restrictive cardiomyopathy (amyloidosis, sarcoidosis, and hemochromatosis)
- Causes of primary right-sided failure include sleep apnea and chronic pulmonary embolism
- MMC Right-sided heart failure is Left-sided heart failure

Clinical Presentation

- Some symptoms include: Exertional dyspnea, Orthopnea, Paroxysmal nocturnal dyspnea, Dyspnea at rest and Acute pulmonary edema

Treatment

- Oxygen
- Vasodilators
- Inotropic agents
- Anticoagulants
- BP lowering medication
- Surgical CABG may be an option if blockage is suspected

Parkinson's Disease

Definition

- Loss of pigmented dopaminergic neurons of the substantia nigra pars compacta
- Presence of Lewy bodies and Lewy neuritis

Clinical Presentation

- Gross resting tremor (pill rolling) of the hands and sometimes feet
- Bradykinesia, rigidity (lead pipe and cogwheeling) and postural instability (unable to maintain balance when pulled from behind)
- Parkinsonian gait (rapid small steps)
- Masked facies, decreased blinking, stooped posture, and salivation

Treatment

- *Clinical diagnosis* and onset is insidious and asymmetric
- A favorable response to levodopa helps confirm the diagnosis

- *Levodopa (L-dopa) + Carbidopa*, a peripheral decarboxylase inhibitor (PDI)
- Deep Brain Stimulation

Pulmonary HTN

Definition

- Elevated pulmonary artery pressure
- 2/3 have right to left shunting across PFO on Echo

Clinical Presentation

- Dyspnea (initially with exertion and then at rest), fatigue, dizziness, syncope, chest pressure or pain, ankle edema
- S3 gallop
- Right ventricular heave
- Pulmonic Regurge (Graham Steele Murmur)

Treatment

- Gold standard test: *Right Heart Catheter*
- Best diagnostic test: TEE (Transesophageal Echocardiogram)
- CCBs
    - Nifedipine
- Encourage healthy diet that is complementary to arterial health
- PDE-5 inhibitors
- Diuretics
- Anticoagulants

Angina

Definition

- Classically described as sub sternal chest pressure or heaviness radiating to the left shoulder and arm, neck, or jaw
- **Stable:** Intensity, character, and frequency of episodes can be predicted; occurs in response to a *known amount of exercise* or other stress state

- **Unstable:** Unpredictable: pain is precipitated by less exercise or has longer duration
    - Angina at rest and new-onset angina, usually >20 min
    - Implies coronary artery plaque instability and is classified as an acute coronary syndrome

- **Variant:** Pain, which can occur at rest
    - Secondary to vasospasm of the coronary arteries
    - Associated with ST segment elevation that resolves with nitroglycerin or CCBs

Clinical Presentation

- SOB, diaphoresis, pain in neck/ shoulder/ arm

Treatment

Stable: occasional NGT

Unstable:

- Admit to telemetry bed
- Serial CEs
- Serial EKGs
- Antiplatelet agents (ASA 325mg or Plavix 300mg)
- Anticoagulation for ongoing pain
- Increase antianginals (nitrates, BBs, CCBs)
- ACEIs, especially in the case of a frank MI

Pericarditis

Definition

- Inflammation of the pericardium
- Causes: viral, associated with renal failure, TB, carcinomatous from breast or lung CA, post-MI, SLE-associated, RA-associated

Clinical Presentation

- Pleuritic chest pain that radiates to shoulder
- Worse when lying down and better when sitting up
- Classic EKG shows *diffuse ST elevation and PR depression*

Treatment

- **After STEMI**: Aspirin is recommended (doses as high as 650mg)
- Colchicine 0.6mg PO q 12 hours
- Anticoagulation should be immediately discontinued if pericardial effusion develops or increases
- Steroids are a last resort
- **MCC Viral/ Inflammatory**: *NSAIDS, especially indomethacin* Consider colchicine 0.6mg PO q 12 hours

Leukemias

Chronic Myelogenous leukemia (CML)

- Many patients are asymptomatic but may present with splenomegaly, weight loss, malaise, bleeding, or thrombosis
- Incidence slowly increases until the *mid-40s* at which point the incidence starts to rise rapidly
- 90% of CML patients have the *Philadelphia chromosome* (translocation of 1/2 of long arm of chromosome 22 to chromosome 9)

Chronic lymphocytic leukemia (CLL)

- CLL is a predominantly malignant clonal disorder of B-lymphocytes.
- There is primary involvement of the bone marrow and secondary release into the peripheral blood

Clinical Presentation

- Usually asymptomatic but can have lymphadenopathy, splenomegaly, and hepatomegaly develop
- *Mean age of diagnosis is 60*
- Chromosomal abnormalities, such as trisomy 12 are common
- Can be caused by damage to the bone marrow from agents such as benzene and ionizing radiation

Acute lymphocytic leukemia (ALL)

Clinical Presentation

- Progressive weakness and fatigue secondary to anemia, infection secondary to leukopenia, and bleeding secondary to thrombocytopenia
- When 50% of the bone marrow is replaced, then peripheral blood cytopenias are observed
- ALL is the *most common malignancy in children*
- Only makes up 20% of adult leukemia's
- The childhood type is more aggressive

Acute Myelogenous leukemia (AML)

Clinical Presentation

- Progressive anemia, leukopenia, and thrombocytopenia
- AML constitutes 15-20% of acute leukemias in children
- The incidence increases with age (significantly higher incidence in those *over age 65*)
- *Auer rods* can be found in AML

PCOS vs. Cushing's

- **Cushing's**: ↑ Cortisol
- **PCOS:** ↑ Androgens/Testosterone
- Both: Can present with weight gain, hirsutism, acne, and irregular periods in women
- Cushing's has easy bruising, sleep disturbances, decreased libido, a buffalo hump, and abdominal striae, which are not present in PCOS
- *The treatment of CS* is primarily the surgical removal of a pituitary, adrenal, or ectopic tumor
- *The treatment for PCOS* is primarily medical and includes oral contraceptives, biguanides (metformin), thiazolidinediones (rosiglitazone or pioglitazone) or androgen antagonists (spirolactone or flutamide)

Testosterone can help differentiate:

- Free Androgen Index (FAI) is low in patients with Cushing's
- Elevated in patients with PCOS

Cushing's:

- Elevated AM fasting cortisol, elevated 24 hr. urine free cortisol
- Dexamethasone suppression test (normal is <2 ug/dL)

Cushing's syndrome is more frequent in women than men, increases age-adjusted and sex-adjusted mortality 5x; yet once identified *can be cured*

PCOS is a heterogeneous disorder that can be *managed but not cured*

Associations

- Cervical Motion Tenderness: "Chandelier sign": **PID**
- Pre-renal cause of ARF: **Cirrhosis**
- Flat, red, well demarcated rash on the inner thigh of a male: **Tinea Cruris**
- 1st line Tx for ischemic cardiomyopathy: **ACE-I**
- MC Congenital Heart disorder: **Bicuspid Aortic Valve** (should be tricuspid in nature)
- **Dressler's Syndrome**: Secondary form of pericarditis, post MI
- Nephrotic Syndrome: **Protein** in the urine
- RA: Type of arthritis that **gets better throughout the day**
- Pericardial Tamponade Tx before paracentesis: **Fluids**
- SLE: **Butterfly Rash**
- Meningitis: **CT first** then- Lumbar puncture as long as no ↑ICP
- DMII 1st Tx: **Metformin**
- Sinus Infection: Nasal Saline Flush (**most are Viral**, so you do not want to Tx with Abx 1st)
- **HCTZ**: 1st Tx for HTN after lifestyle changes, if not contraindicated
- Most specific test for TB: **Sputum Culture**
- Decompensated Cirrhosis: **Ascites**
- Wernicke-Korsakoff syndrome: **Thiamine (B1)**
- Major depression >**2 weeks**

Chapter Four

Pediatrics

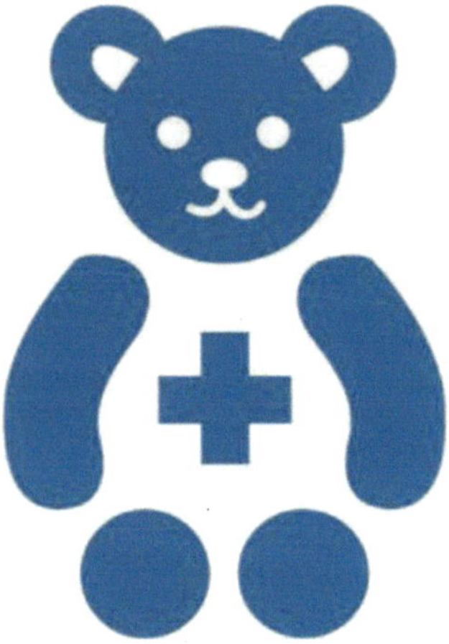

Milestones

- Sit unsupported: ***6 mos.***
- Stand/babbles momma/dada: ***9 mos.***
- Walk: *12 mos.*

Physical Abuse

Common fracture seen in children being abused

- Spiral fractures; if seen look for other signs of abuse.
- Shaken baby syndrome: can cause contusion on the brain, brain swelling and death.

Who is most likely to be the abuser: *mother's boyfriend.*

Apgar Score

	0 Points	1 Point	2 Points	Total
Activity (Muscle Tone)	Absent	Arms and legs Flexed	Active Movement	
Pulse	Absent	Below 100	Over 100 bpm	
Grimace (Reflex Irritability)	Flaccid	Some Flexion of Extremities	Active motion (coughing, pull away)	
Appearance	Blue, Pale	Body is pink and Extremities Blue	Completely Pink	
Respiration	Absent	Slow, Irregular	Vigorously Crying	

Severely Depressed: 0-3 (Below 3, patient will need to be intubated)
Moderately Depressed: 4-6
Excellent Condition: 7-10

High Bilirubin

Jaundice

- Jaundice is the *most common condition that requires medical attention in newborns*
- Jaundice is the result of *accumulation of unconjugated bilirubin*
- An excessive rise can be cause for concern because unconjugated bilirubin is *neurotoxic* and can cause death in newborns and lifelong neurologic sequelae in infants who survive (*kernicterus*)

Kernicterus

- Bilirubin staining can be noted on autopsy in the basal ganglia, hippocampus, substantia nigra, and brainstem nuclei
- Factors influencing permeability of the blood-brain barrier (acidosis, infection) and the amount of unbound (versus albumin-bound) bilirubin
- Bilirubin often accumulates in the gray matter
- Infants are more susceptible because the blood brain barrier is not fully developed
- Treatment with sunlight may help; no other medical treatment

Polycythemia

Definition

- Abnormally *increased concentration of hemoglobin* in the blood, through either reduction of plasma volume or increase in red cell number
- Maternal smoking, maternal illness, placental insufficiency, and gestation at high altitude, can result in neonatal polycythemia
- Delayed clamping of the cord, stripping the cord, or holding the baby below the level of the introitus for a prolonged period, can result in increased RBC mass in the baby
- This is particularly true for babies born in the absence of a trained birth attendant

Hemolysis

Definition

- Destruction of Red Blood Cells (RBC)
- *Immune hemolytic disease*, most often Rh isoimmunization (erythroblastosis fetalis), is the prototype etiology for kernicterus
- *ABO iso-immunization*, as well as minor blood group antigens, can also cause hemolytic disease in the newborn
- *Membrane defects*, such as hereditary spherocytosis and elliptocytosis; enzyme defects, such as glucose-6-phosphate dehydrogenase deficiency and pyruvate kinase deficiency; and hemoglobinopathies, such as alpha and beta thalassemias can predispose the infant to hemolysis

Sickle cell disease does *not typically* cause hemolytic disease in the neonatal period

Some Causes of Hemolytic Anemia

Hereditary Spherocytosis	Sphere shaped rather than bi-concave RBC's
Elliptocytosis	RBC's that are elliptical shaped
G6PD	(favism) (Fava Bean) decreased G6PD with is important in the function of the Pentose Phosphate Pathway and is also protective against malaria
PKD	A metabolic disorder, which causes a decreased in the amount of ATP made in RBC's

Cephalohematoma and Caput Succedaneum

Cephalohematoma

- **Sub periosteal** collection of blood caused by rupture of vessels *beneath the peri-osteum* (usually over the parietal or occipital bone)

- A present as swelling that does *not cross suture lines*. Calcification can occur
- Resolve in 2 wks. -3 mos
- Usually occurs from prolonged Labor, Vacuum Extraction, and forceps delivery

Caput Succedaneum

- Edematous **swelling of the scalp above the periosteum**, which is occasionally hemorrhagic
- It presents at birth after prolonged engagement of the fetal head in the birth canal or after vacuum extraction
- Unlike Cephalohematoma, it *extends across the suture lines*.
- Caput succedaneum is generally a benign condition, and it usually resolves within a few days and requires no treatment

ADHD

3 types of attention deficit hyperactivity disorder (ADHD)

- Predominantly hyperactive
- Predominantly inattentive
- Combined

Criteria

- Onset is no later than age *7 years*
- Symptoms must be present in *2 or more situations*, such as school, work, or home
- The disturbance causes clinically *significant distress* or *impairment* in social, academic, or occupational functioning
- Disorder does not occur exclusively during the course of a pervasive developmental disorder, schizophrenia, or other psychotic disorder and is not better accounted for by mood, anxiety, dissociative, or personality disorder

Treatment

- Psychotherapy and Behavioral therapy
- Amphetamine Salts (methylphenidate)

Intussusception

Definition

- Intussusception is where a segment of intestine invaginates into the adjoining intestinal lumen, causing bowel obstruction
- With early diagnosis, appropriate fluid resuscitation, and therapy, the mortality rate from intussusception in children is less than 1%
- If left untreated, however, this condition is uniformly fatal in 2-5 days

Symptoms

- Sudden, crampy abdominal pain in which patient draws legs to chest
- *Currant jelly stools*
- **Vomiting:** Initially, vomiting is non-bilious and reflexive, but when the intestinal obstruction occurs, vomiting becomes bilious
- **Abdominal pain**: Pain in intussusception is *colicky, severe, and intermittent*
- **Passage of blood and mucus:** Parents report the passage of stools, by affected children, that look like *currant jelly*; this is a mixture of mucus, sloughed mucosa, and shed blood; diarrhea can also be an early sign of intussusception
- **Lethargy:** This can be the sole presenting symptom of intussusception, which makes the condition's diagnosis challenging
- **Palpable abdominal mass** ("*Sausage like mass*")

Imaging: Barium Enema can be *therapeutic and diagnostic*. Surgery is the last option, which can lead to *short gut syndrome*.

Pyloric Stenosis

Definition

- Narrowing (*stenosis*) of the duodenum, due to enlargement (*hypertrophy*) of the muscle surrounding the pylorus, which spasms when the stomach empties

Symptoms

Projectile vomiting usually in first 2-3 mos. of life

- Infantile hypertrophic pyloric stenosis (IHPS) is the most common cause of intestinal obstruction in infancy
- IHPS occurs secondary to hypertrophy and hyperplasia of the muscular layers of the pylorus, causing a functional gastric outlet obstruction

Classic: *Pyloric stenosis has non-bilious vomiting or regurgitation, which may become projectile (in asmany as 70% of cases), after which the infant is still hungry*

- Emesis may be intermittent or occur after each feeding
- The emesis may become brown or coffee color due to blood secondary to gastritis or a Mallory-Weiss tear at the gastro-esophageal junction
- The infant begins to show signs of dehydration and malnutrition, such as: poor weight gain, weight loss, marasmus, decreased urinary output, lethargy, and shock
- The infant may develop jaundice, which is corrected upon correction of the disease

Treatment

- *Surgical correction* is considered the *standard of care*
- Immediate treatment requires correction of fluid loss, electrolytes, and acid-base imbalance
- The dehydrated infant should receive an initial bolus (20 mL/kg) of crystalloid fluid
- The infant should remain nothing by mouth (*NPO*)

#1 Risk factor Asthma = Atopy

Definition

Predisposition toward developing certain allergic hypersensitivity reactions.

- **Signs of Atopy**
  - Eczema
  - Atopic Dermatitis
  - Allergic Rhinitis

Peritonsillar Abscess

Definition

- *Unilateral swelling* of the peritonsillar area
- Unilateral swelling of the soft palate, with *anterior displacement* of the ipsilateral tonsil
- No resolution of acute tonsillitis, with persistent unilateral tonsillar enlargement

Clinical Presentation

- Have unilateral pharyngeal asymmetry, dehydration and can be septic
- *Uvula shifted to contralateral side of abscess*
- Most patients have severe pain

Examination

- Marked erythema in mouth, asymmetry of the soft palate, tonsillar exudation, and contralateral displacement of the uvula

Workup

- PA and Lateral of Neck, CT scan and Ultrasound

Diagnostic Procedure

- *Needle aspiration of the abscess* and drainage
- This allows identification of the location of the abscess in the peritonsillar space

Treatment

- High dose PCN or Cephalexin or other cephalosporin (with or without metronidazole)

Alternatives include the following

- Cefuroxime or cefpodoxime (with or without metronidazole)
- Clindamycin
- Trovafloxacin
- Amoxicillin-clavulanate (if mononucleosis has been ruled out)
- Oral antibiotics may be prescribed once the patient is able to tolerate oral intake
- *Treatment should be continued for 7-10 days*

Bronchiolitis

Definition

- This is an acute inflammatory injury of the bronchioles that is usually caused by a viral infection
- MC: *Respiratory Syncytial Virus* (60%)
- *Human Metapneumovirus*
- This is generally a *clinical diagnosis*

Bronchiolitis is most common in children *less than 2 years old*.

Clinical Presentation

- Infants may become increasingly fussy and have difficulty feeding during a 2 to 5-day incubation period
- Symptoms include development of cough, dyspnea, wheezing, and feeding difficulties and in infants < 1 month can present as hypothermia
- A low-grade fever, usually less than 101.5°F, and increasing coryza and congestion usually follow the incubation period

Physical Exam

- Tachypnea, nasal flaring, retractions, irritability, and, possibly, cyanosis

Workup

- CBC, pulse ox
- Possible workup for sepsis
- Viral culture for RSV
- Chest X-ray: show lobar infiltrates or atelectasis or both

Treatment

- Remove offending agent (chemical inhalants, smoke)
- Hydration
- Suction for access mucus
- Symptomatic relief

Croup

Definition

- Primarily a pediatric viral respiratory tract illness
- Croup primarily affects the larynx and trachea, which makes it a URI

Clinical Presentation

- Can manifest as hoarseness, "*seal-like barking cough*", inspiratory stridor, and a variable degree of respiratory distress
- Morbidity is secondary to narrowing of the larynx and trachea below the level of the glottis (subglottic region), causing an inspiratory stridor

Imaging

- X-ray: *Steeple sign*

Treatment

- **Mild**: Take a hot shower followed immediately by cool air or mist
- **Severe**: The anti-inflammatory action of *corticosteroids* reduces laryngeal mucosal edema and decreases the need for salvage-nebulized epinephrine
- *Nebulized racemic epinephrine* or *L-epinephrine* is typically reserved for patients in moderate to severe distress
    - Epinephrine constricts the precapillary arterioles through adrenergic stimulation, thereby decreasing capillary hydrostatic pressure
    - This leads to fluid resorption from the interstitium and improvement in the laryngeal mucosal edema

If stridor at rest

- Racemic epinephrine immediately
- Corticosteroids: dexamethasone IM or PO 1 dose

Epiglottitis

Definition

- An acute inflammation in the supraglottic region of the oropharynx with inflammation of the epiglottis, vallecula, arytenoids, and aryepiglottic folds
- *"Thumbprint sign"* ***on lateral Neck***

Clinical Presentation

- Common in children *2-4 yrs. old*
- Associated upper airway obstruction has significant morbidity and mortality and may cause respiratory arrest and death

Treatment

- MC it is a polymicrobial infection in nature
    - Give broad spectrum Abx such as Ceftriaxone, Cefotaxime or Unasyn and get blood cultures, as *25% of pts are Septic*
    - Laryngoscopy is recommended before extubation
    - Since the *introduction of the Hib vaccine* and the accompanying dramatic reduction in H influenza type b invasive disease incidence, epiglottitis has become *rare in children*

Treatment should continue for *7-10 days*

Otitis Externa

Definition

- Otitis Externa (OE) or (Swimmers Ear) is an inflammation or infection of the external auditory canal (EAC), the auricle, or both. This condition can be found in all age groups.

Clinical Presentation

- Discharge is common
- Acute bacterial infection of the skin of the ear canal
- MC: *Pseudomonas Aeruginosis or Staphylococcus aureus*

Acute diffuse OE

- Most common form of OE: typically seen in swimmers
- *Rapid onset* (generally within 48 hours)
- Symptoms of EAC inflammation (such as: Otalgia, itching, or fullness, with or without hearing loss or jaw pain) as well as tenderness of the tragus or pinna or diffuse ear edema or erythema or both, with or without otorrhea, regional lymphadenitis, tympanic membrane erythema, or cellulitis of the pinna

Treatment

- **Topical:** Hydrocortisone/neomycin/polymyxin is an antibacterial and anti-inflammatory agent for otic use, available as a solution or a suspension
- **Oral:** Cipro for infection or cellulitis

Fluoroquinolones are the drugs of choice by virtue of their coverage of Pseudomonas species.

Acute Otitis Media

Definition

- The middle ear shows signs and symptoms of acute inflammation
- MC affliction necessitating medical therapy for children younger than 5 years old

Clinical Presentation

Neonates	Irritability or feeding difficulties may be the only indication of a septic focus
Older children	This age group begins to demonstrate a consistent presence of fever and otalgia, or ear tugging
Older children and adults	Hearing loss becomes a constant feature of AOM and otitis media with effusion (OME); ear stuffiness is noted before the detection of middle ear fluid

Physical Exam

- Tympanic membrane of a person with ***12 hours of ear pain****, slight tympanic membrane bulge, and slight meniscus of purulent effusion* at bottom of tympanic membrane

- Pneumatic otoscopy: Best tool for differentiating AOM from acute bullous myringitis. The latter condition, in its purest form, manifests ***10-14 days*** after a viral infection and causes severe localized Otalgia without middle ear effusion

Treatment: *Amoxicillin or Augmentin*

Streptococcal Pharyngitis

Definition: Centor Criteria

- A recent fever of 101 °F (38.3 °C) or higher
- White or yellow spots or coating on the throat or tonsils
- Swollen or tender lymph nodes on the neck
- Absence of signs of a cold or upper respiratory infection, such as coughing or sneezing

Testing

- **Rapid strep test**: Analyzes the bacteria in your throat to see if strep is the cause of your sore throat
- **Throat culture:** This test analyzes cell samples from the back of your throat

Treatment

- *Penicillin or Amoxicillin (First line)*
- Cephalosporin (Strong evidence)
- Azithromycin (Moderate evidence)

Scarlett Fever presentation

Definition

- A syndrome characterized by *exudative pharyngitis, fever, and bright-red exanthema*
- It is caused by a toxin-producing bacterium*: Group A-beta-hemolytic streptococci (GABHS)* found in secretions and discharge from the nose, ears, throat, and skin
- Scarlet fever may follow streptococcal wound infections or burns, as well as URIs

Treatment

Goals

- *Prevent acute rheumatic fever*
- Reduce the spread of infection
- *Prevent post streptococcal glomerulonephritis and suppurative sequelae* Such as: (adenitis, mastoiditis, ethmoiditis, abscesses, and cellulitis)
- Shorten the course of illness.
- **Abx**: *PCN* unless allergic- otherwise: *Erythromycin* is the drug of choice

PSGN

Definition

- Acute glomerulonephritis: *sudden appearance of hematuria, proteinuria, red blood cell casts in the urine, edema, and hypertension with or without oliguria*
- It can follow streptococcal infections that are not treated
    - Recognized complication of scarlet fever

Clinical Presentation

- *A latent period always occurs* between strep and glomerulonephritis that is *1-2 weeks after a throat infection and 3-6 weeks after a skin infection*
- The onset of signs and symptoms at the **same time** as pharyngitis (also called Synpharyngitic Nephritis) = Immunoglobulin A (IgA) nephropathy rather than APSGN

Dark urine: (*Cola-colored*) is often the *first clinical manifestation* of APSGN. Dark urine is caused by hemolysis of red blood cells that have penetrated the glomerular basement membrane and have passed into the tubular system

Physical Exam

- *Periorbital edema is typical.* The onset is sudden and usually prominent upon awakening and, if the patient is active
- Tends to subside at the end of the day

Treatment

- Symptomatic treatment: The major aims are to:
    - *Control the edema and blood pressure*
- During the acute phase of the disease, *salt and water should be restricted*
- Antibiotic therapy is the treatment of choice for scarlet fever

Ventricle Septal Defect (VSD)

Definition

- A hole or a *defect in the septum* that divides the 2 lower chambers of the heart
- This is a left to right shunt. (Non-cyanotic)

Clinical Presentation

Small: Mild or no symptoms
Moderate: Fatigue with feeding
Large: Poor weight gain and increased incidence of respiratory infections

This is the *most common congenital heart defect.*

Imaging

- Echocardiography is used for surgical closure
- Cardiac catheterization is used for a moderate to large septal defect, or for pulmonary hypertension

Treatment

- *Surgical repair* is indicated in older asymptomatic children with a normal pulmonary pressure if the pulmonary-to-systemic flow ratio (Qp:Qs) is greater than 2:1
- *Prolapse of an aortic valve cusp* is an indication for surgery even if the VSD is small
    - Early repair may prevent progression of the aortic insufficiency

Medications: Diuretics, angiotensin-converting enzyme (ACE) inhibitors, and cardiac glycosides to control symptoms of CHF.

Coarctation of aorta

Definition

- The word "Coarctation" means *narrowing*
- MC where the aorta arches toward the abdomen and legs

- Coarctation of the aorta (CoA) is a relatively common defect that accounts for 5-8% of all congenital heart defects
- Coarctation of the aorta may occur in association with various other lesions, MC *bicuspid aortic valve* and *ventricular septal defect (VSD)*

Clinical Presentation

- Diagnosis is often delayed until the patient develops *congestive heart failure* (CHF), which is common in infants, or *hypertension*, which is common in older children
- Aortic Coarctation is considered when a *section of the aorta is narrowed to an abnormal width*

Treatment

- Significant hypertension or congestive heart failure (CHF) is an indication for intervention
- If neither hypertension nor heart failure is present, elective surgical or balloon therapy in children aged 2-5 years is suggested
- Operative mortality rates:
    - Neonates and infants: (4-50%)
    - Older children: (0-5%)

Patent Ductus Arteriosis (PDA)

Definition

- A persistent communication between the descending thoracic aorta and the pulmonary artery that results from failure of normal physiologic closure of the fetal ductus

Clinical Presentation

- Three-week to 6-week-old infants can present with tachypnea, diaphoresis, inability or difficulty with feeding, and weight loss or no weight gain
- A ductus arteriosus with a moderate-to-large left-to-right shunt may be associated with a hoarse cry, cough, lower respiratory tract infections, atelectasis, or pneumonia

Physical Exam: "*Machine like murmur*"

- A *widened pulse pressure* and *suprasternal or carotid pulsations present.*
- Apical impulse is laterally displaced
- Thrill may be present in the suprasternal notch or in the left infraclavicular region
- Several clicks may be heard that sounds like "*shaking dice*" or "*shaking a bag of rocks*"

Imaging

- CXR ranges from normal to those consistent for congestive heart failure (CHF)
- EKG: *T-wave inversion* and *ST segment depression* may be present, suggesting ischemia or a supply-demand mismatch

Treatment

- Respiratory distress or impaired systemic oxygen delivery is sign that treatment is needed
- Give *Intravenous (IV) indomethacin* within first 10-14 days of life
- *Surgical ligation or surgical ligation and division* are needed for a large (PDA) that requires treatment in infancy

Phimosis

Definition

- The inability to retract the distal foreskin over the glans penis
- Physiologic phimosis occurs naturally in newborn males
- Pathologic phimosis is usually due to *distal scarring of the foreskin*
  - This is rarely a urological emergency

Treatment

- The use of *soaking in an osmotic solution* for 2 hours before *manual reduction* is helpful
- A 20-gauge needle can be used to *aspirate 3-12 mL of blood* from the glans, parallel to the urethra
- *Emergent circumcision is the last resort*

Paraphimosis

Definition

- Entrapment of a retracted foreskin behind the coronal sulcus.
- Paraphimosis is a disease of uncircumcised or partially circumcised males
    - *Paraphimosis is a urologic emergency* and needs to be attended to immediately

Treatment

- Manual reduction, puncture method (up to 20 punctures), immediate circumcision and aspiration

Hydrocele

Definition

- A hydrocele is a fluid collection within the tunica vaginalis of the scrotum or along the spermatic cord

Clinical Presentation

- *Painless swelling* of fluid in processes vaginalis/tunica, commonly resolves without intervention within one year
    - May need surgery if still they don't resolve in one year

- **Non-communicating:** Fluid cannot flow back and forth into abdomen when supine
- **Communicating**: Enlarges with upright position and lessens with supine position or compression

Physical Exam

- Typically manifest as a *soft non-tender fullness within the hemi-scrotum*
- The testis is generally palpable along the posterior aspect of the fluid collection
- When the scrotum is investigated with a focused beam of light, the *scrotum trans illuminates*, revealing a homogenous glow, without internal shadows

Treatment

- Surgical inguinal approach with *ligation of the processus vaginalis* high within the internal inguinal ring is treatment of choice for pediatric hydroceles (typically, communicating)

Testicular Torsion

Definition

- Acute scrotal pain, sudden twisting of testicle on blood supply
- MC during puberty and in newborns
- It is common for the attachment of the tunica vaginalis to the testicle to be inappropriately high; the spermatic cord can rotate within it, which can lead to intravaginal torsion

Clinical Presentation

- "*Bell Clapper Deformity*" happens in about 17% of males and is bilateral in 40%. Intra-vaginal testicular torsion produces a *sudden onset of severe unilateral scrotal pain* followed by inguinal and/or scrotal swelling
- Pain may lessen with necrosis- especially seen in newborns
- Symptoms include *gastrointestinal upset* with *nausea and vomiting*

Imaging: Ultrasound/ Nuclear scans and blood flow doppler.

Treatment

- ***Emergency***: Treat w/ immediate surgery within 6 hours
- Surgical de-torsion is the definitive treatment for testicular torsion
    - This must be done to avoid Orchidoplexy

Appendage torsion

Definition

- This is a twisting of the appendages or tail of the epididymis.
- 92% of all testes and is usually located at the *superior testicular pole* in the groove between the testicle and the epididymis

Two appendages

- **Appendix testis:** A remnant of the paramesonephric (müllerian) duct
- **Appendix epididymis:** A remnant of the mesonephric (wolffian) duct

Clinical Presentation

- *Gradual onset*
- Pain is MC in the upper pole of the testicle
- *Nausea and vomiting are usually not associated with this condition*

Physical Exam

- The testis should be *non-tender to palpation* and there is usually a para-testicular nodule at the superior aspect of the testicle
  - Characteristic "*blue-dot*" appearance in 21% of cases

Treatment

- *NSAIDs and ice* are the mainstays of therapy for inflammation
- Pain may last 1-3 weeks and then resolve

Urinary Tract Infection

Definition

- A UTI is an infection in the urogenital system including the bladder, urethra or kidneys
- MC *pediatric infection*
- The workup of fever in these infants should always include evaluation for UTI

Clinical Presentation

Neonates with UTI may display the following symptoms

- Jaundice, Fever, Failure to thrive, Poor feeding, Vomiting, Irritability

Clinical Presentation

- In 2-24 month old, presence of pyuria and/or bacteriuria on urinalysis and at least 50,000 colony-forming units (CFU) per mL of a uropathogen from the quantitative culture of a properly collected urine specimen

Labs

- Urine Specimen, UA, CBC, Creatine/ BUN

Imaging

- Ultrasound

Treatment

- Oral empiric antibiotics (Ceftriaxone, Ampicillin, Augmentin) for coverage of the most common uropathogens
  - MC *Escherichia coli* and *Enterococcus, Proteus, and Klebisella species*

For recurring UTI: *Bactrim*

Anemia

Definition

- A reduction in the number of circulating red blood cells (RBCs), the amount of hemoglobin, or the volume of packed red blood cells (hematocrit)

Labs

- The most important index is the mean corpuscular volume (*MCV*). This is to classify the anemia as microcytic, normocytic, or macrocytic

Microcytic: MCV <80	Anemias of chronic disease, iron deficiency, lead poisoning, and the hemoglobinopathies (such as; sickle cell disease, sideroblastic anemia, thalassemias)
Normocytic: MCV 80-100	Acute blood loss, hemolysis, uremia, and cancer
Macrocytic: MCV >100	Alcoholism, folate and vitamin B-12 deficiencies (pernicious anemia)

Bilirubin/ BUN: Rule out GI bleed

Reticulocyte count: Suggests an inadequate bone marrow response to anemia. Can rule out aplastic anemia, hematologic cancer, drugs or toxins.

PT/ aPTT: To rule out DIC

Beta-HCG: To rule out pregnancy

Iron Studies

Folate

Hemoglobin electrophoresis

Blood Smear

Treatment

- Restore hemodynamics, hemoglobin and RBC's. The use of mineral and vitamin supplements, blood transfusions, vasopressors, histamine (H2) antagonists, and glucocorticosteroids are acceptable

Cerebral palsy

Definition

- An "umbrella" term describing *non-progressive brain lesions involving motor or postural abnormalities* that are noted during early development
- Leading cause of childhood disability affecting function and development

Clinical Presentation

- Manifests as *early hypotonia* for the first 6 months to 1 year of life, followed by *spasticity*. *Abnormal muscle tone*

The most frequently observed symptoms

- *Growth disturbance*: Especially failure to thrive
- *Increased reflexes*: Indicating the presence of an upper motor neuron lesion

Other manifestations include

- Mental retardation
- Ophthalmologic and hearing impairments
- Speech and language disorders
- Oromotor dysfunction

Labs

Thyroid function tests
Lactate and pyruvate
Anomia levels Chromosomal
analysis Cerebrospinal
protein levels

CT Scan: Shows enlarged ventricles, cystic encephalomalacia and decreased white matter

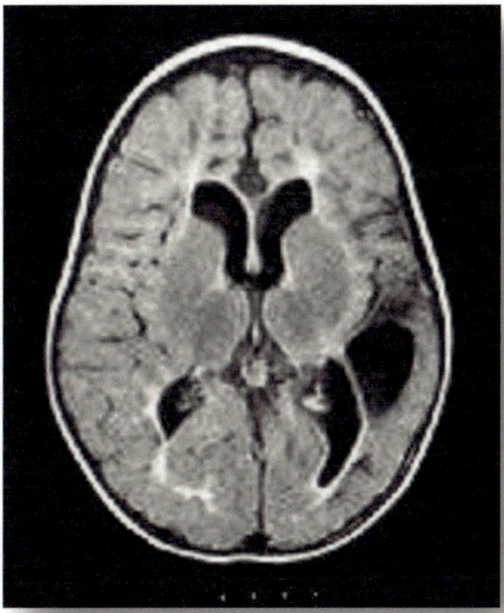

Figure 4: MRI of 16-month-old boy with anoxic event at delivery.
Source: http://emedicine.medscape.com/article/1179555-overview

Treatment

- Medications such as: Anti-parkinsonian, anticonvulsant, anti-dopaminergic, and antidepressant agents are acceptable

Febrile Seizure

Definition

- A fever (101.4) or above associated with a seizure. Fever in a child aged *6 months to 5 years* is MC

This is the MC type of seizure observed in the pediatric age group

Two Types

- **Simple febrile seizures** (which are generalized, last < 15 min and do not recur within 24 h)
- **Complex febrile seizures** (which are prolonged, recur more than once in 24 h, or are focal)

Clinical Presentation

- Viral illnesses such as *human herpes simplex virus 6 (HHSV-6)* is the MC etiologic agent in roseola in about 20% of a group of patients presenting with their first febrile seizures
- *Shigella gastroenteritis* also has been associated with febrile seizures

Treatment: Rectal Diazepam

Epilepsy

Definition

- Enduring ability for the brain to generate epileptic seizures by the neurobiological, cognitive, psychological, and social consequences of this condition

Labs

- *Prolactin levels* obtained shortly after a seizure to assess the etiology (*epileptic vs. non-epileptic pseudo-seizures*)
    - Levels are typically elevated 3 or 4-fold and more likely to occur with generalized tonic-clonic seizures.
- EEG, MRI, CT

Treatment

- *Anticonvulsants* such as (Clobazam, Carbamazepine or lamotrigine) for patients at increased risk of re-occurrence

Primary Generalized Tonic-Clonic Seizures

Definition

- Tonic-clonic seizures or "*grand mal seizures*". They consist of several motor behaviors; such as generalized *tonic extension of the extremities* lasting for few seconds *followed by clonic rhythmic movements* and *prolonged postictal confusion*

Clinical Presentation

- Partial seizure: Typically has no aura
- Secondary generalized tonic-clonic seizures: Has an aura
- The aura preceding the partial seizure with secondary generalization is often forgotten because of postictal amnesia

Labs

- **EEG:** *The Ictal correlate* consists of *generalized (bilateral) complexes of spikes or poly-spike and slow waves on EEG*
- These epileptiform discharges often have increased amplitude in the frontal regions

Treatment

- *Anticonvulsants* such as (Clobazam, Carbamazepine or lamotrigine) for risk of re-occurrence
- Most who have a primary seizure will never have a seizure again

Developmental dysplasia of hip

Definition

- Abnormal development of the hip which may include the acetabulum and the proximal femur, as well as the labrum, capsule, and other soft tissues

Physical Exam

- **Barlow (dislocation)**: Apply pressure with thumb on medial side of thigh as it is adducted
  - Slipping of hip posteriorly will *elicit a jerk* as the hip dislocates

- **Ortolani (reduction)**: Both hips flexed to 90 degrees, slowly abducted from midline, gentle pressure in attempt to lift greater trochanter forward
  - Feeling a *slipping/clunk and audible click* as head relocates; this is indicative of *instability*

Treatment

- *Bilateral hip dislocation* in a patient without false acetabula has a *better overall prognosis*
- Open reduction for children who are older than 2 years at the time of the initial diagnosis

Legg-Calve-Perthes-Disease

Definition

- LCPD is *avascular necrosis* of capital epiphysis of femoral head resulting from the compromise of the tenuous blood supply to this area and usually happens between the ages of 4-10yrs old
- A *slipped capital femoral epiphysis* is the displacement of femoral head on femoral neck

Imaging: X-Ray

Treatment

- Minimize pain and surgical innominate osteotomy
- A femoral osteotomy may cause shortening of the limb and a chronic limp

Nursemaid's Elbow

Definition

- This is a radial head subluxation, also known as "*pulled elbow*"
- This is the *MC upper-extremity injury* in infants and young children <6 yrs. Old who present to the emergency department

Clinical Presentation

- Child not using affected arm and holding it close to body and has pain

Treatment

- Provide analgesics for pain.
- Pull the forearm while it is pronated and the elbow is extended at the same time
- This results in reduction of the radial head
    - Instruct patents not to pull on the child's arm

Scaphoid fracture

Definition

- Fall on outstretched hand, pain at snuffbox, worry about avascular necrosis
- Thumb spica

Imaging

- All wrist injuries should include *4 views*
    - Poster anterior (PA), lateral, and supinated and pronated obliques
    - All patients should also have a view of the scaphoid/ Navicular bone because the scaphoid is fractured *71%* MC out of all carpel bones
    - The PA view on radiograph should be taken with the *wrist extended 30° and deviated ulnarly 20°*

Treatment

- Immobilization in a *thumb Spica cast for 2 weeks* (allowing for resorption at the fracture site)
- *Re-evaluation with repeat radiography*
- Surgery is indicated to prevent necrosis if blood flow to the scaphoid is compromised

Scoliosis

Definition

- Scoliosis is a sideward (right or left) curve in the spine and is a complex, 3-dimensional deformity that often develops in childhood

Treatment

Surgery is indicated in a child that has a *>60 degree* curve

- Scoliosis curves with an RVAD of <20°, observation every 4-6 months is sufficient
- If the RVAD > 20° or if it is *not flexible* clinically (curve cannot be corrected even slightly with different postures, especially lateral bending), then it is considered to be *progressive* until proven otherwise
- Scoliosis < 30 degrees tends not to get worse, while those curves > 50 degrees can get worse over time, by about 1 to 1 1/2 degrees per year

Needs bracing: Curves measuring *25 to 50 degrees* are considered large enough to require bracing

Needs surgery: Curves >50 degrees will likely need surgery to restore normal posture

Impetigo

Definition

- *MC bacterial infection in children*
- Highly contagious infection of the superficial layers of the epidermis
- Caused by *Streptococcus pyogenes* or *Staphylococcus aureus*

Clinical Presentation

- This usually presents as *multiple coalescing lesions* on the face (perioral, perinasal) and extremities
- The lesions are small vesicles or pustules (< 2 cm) that rupture and become a "*honey-colored crust"* with a *moist erythematous base*
- Non-bullous impetigo resolves in 2 weeks

Treatment

- Gentle cleansing and removal of the honey-colored crusts of non-bullous impetigo using antibacterial soap and a washcloth, and frequent application of wet dressings is standard care
- Antibacterial washes, such as *chlorhexidine* or *sodium hypochlorite baths*

- Empiric bacterial coverage is indicated to eradicating Staphylococcus aureus and Group-A Beta-Hemolytic Streptococci (GABHS) such as (*Augmentin, Clindamycin or Erythromycin*)

Pityriasis Rosea

Definition

- Pityriasis Rosea is a *common skin disorder* observed most frequently children and young adults. It is a self-limiting, papulo-squamous eruption that has duration of 6-8 weeks
  - *Secondary syphilis and primary HIV must be ruled out*

Physical Exam

- Disease typically begins with a solitary patch, usually *salmon-colored*, that precedes the eruption of a rash *commonly referred to as the "herald patch/ Christmas tree pattern"*

Labs

- CBC, ESR, Total Serum Protein, Albumin, Rheumatoid Factor,
- Potassium hydrochloride (KOH): To rule out Tinea Corporis
- RPR, VRDL: To rule out Syphilis
- HIV

Treatment

- Treatment is supportive: Water, sweat, and soap may cause irritation
- In severe cases: *Topical Steroids*, *Ultraviolet (UV) radiation* and *topical zinc oxide* and *calamine lotion* are useful for pruritus

Erysipelas

Definition

- "***St. Anthony's fire***" is an acute infection typically with a skin rash, usually on any of the legs and toes, face, arms and fingers
- It is an *infection of the upper dermis and superficial lymphatics* caused by *Beta-Hemolytic Group A Streptococcus*

Clinical Presentation

- **Prodrome**: Malaise, chills, and high fever, begin before the onset of the skin lesions and occur within 48 hours of skin involvement
- Other symptoms include muscle and joint pain, nausea and headache

Labs

- ESR, CRP

Treatment

- Symptomatic relief and prompt treatment is crucial because of rapid progression
- *Penicillin has remained a first-line therapy*. If patient has a PCN allergy, use a first-generation cephalosporin or macrolide, such as erythromycin or azithromycin

Scabies

Definition

- An intensely pruritic skin infestation caused by the host-specific mite *Sarcoptes scabiei hominis*

Clinical Presentation

- *Burrows* are a pathognomonic sign and represent the *intraepidermal tunnel* created by the moving female mite. They appear as *serpiginous, grayish, threadlike elevations* in the superficial epidermis, ranging from 2-10 mm long

Common locations for burrows include the following

- Webbed spaces of the fingers, Flexor surfaces of the wrists, Elbows, Axillae, Belt line, Feet, Scrotum (men) and Areolae in (women)

Treatment

- Standard treatment: Topical scabicidal agents (*Permethrin 5% lotion*) with repeat application in 7 days.

Kawasaki Disease

Definition

- This is a primary systemic vasculitis that is MC in boys, high risk of development of coronary artery aneurysms

Clinical Presentation

- Cough, diarrhea, rhinorrhea, weakness and joint pain
- Possible history of Infectious Mononucleosis

Criteria

5 days of fever (*Must have*)

(+)

4 of the following

- Unilateral Lymphadenopathy (75%): cervical node MC
- Rash
- Injected Conjunctiva (90%)
- Swelling of extremities
- Strawberry tongue/ or mucosal findings
- Groin Swelling (70%)

Treatment

- High Dose Aspirin, IV IgG
- If IVIG-resistant, treat with methotrexate or cyclophosphamide

Mumps

Definition

- Acute, self-limited, systemic viral illness characterized by the swelling of one or more of the salivary glands and MC the *parotid glands*.
- Caused by the RNA virus; Rubulavirus. *Rubulavirus is within the genus Paramyxovirus*

Clinical Presentation

- Fever, headache, and malaise

- Within 24 hours, ear pain localized near the ear lobe and swelling of the mandibular angle is common
- *Orchitis occurs in up to 50%* of post pubertal males

Labs

- CBC, ESR, IgG and IgM titers
- *Nasopharyngeal* or *blood cultures* can isolate the mumps virus, which can be found within 7 days before and up until 9 days after the onset of parotitis

Treatment

- *Supportive care* and isolation is imperative for up to 5 days from the onset of symptoms as well as *adequate hydration*
- Pain can be relieved by *acetaminophen and ibuprofen* as well as cold packs

Roseola Infantum (6th disease)

Definition

- Common childhood disease.
- *Causative organism is Human Herpes Virus: HHV6*

Clinical Presentation

- Affects 9- to 12-month-old infants who acutely develop a high fever and often a febrile seizure (15%).
- After 3 days, a morbilliform rash appears

Labs

- CBC, urinalysis, blood cultures and cerebrospinal fluid exam
- Serologic assay can test for human herpes virus (HHV)–6A- and HHV-6B

Treatment

- No antiviral treatment available

Erythema Infectiosum (5th Disease)

Definition

- Erythema Infectiosum is usually a benign childhood condition characterized by a classic *slapped-cheek appearance* and *lacy exanthem*
- Infection with human parvovirus (PV) B19 that is an erythrovirus

Clinical Presentation

- The *incubation period is 4-14 days* and is *spread via aerosolized respiratory droplets*
- May have prodromal symptoms at approximately 1 week after exposure and last 2-3 days

Symptoms

SYMPTOM	Rate of occurrence in pediatric patients
Headache	20%
Fever	20%
Sore throat	15%
Pruritus	15%
Coryza	10%
Abdominal pain	10%
Arthralgia's	10%

Treatment

- **Primarily symptomatic relief**: IVIG, NSAIDS
- **Severe**: Transfusion for aplastic crisis

Measles

Definition

- Acute infection caused by the rubeola virus
- *Highly contagious* and belongs to the genus *Morbillivirus* of the family Paramyxoviridae

Clinical Presentation

- Classic triad of *cough, coryza (watery nasal discharge), and conjunctivitis*
- *Koplik spots*: White lesions on the buccal mucosa, may be seen 1-2d before the onset of rash
- The *rash is generalized*, erythematous, and maculopapular, appearing 4-7d after symptoms begin and lasting up to 5-7d

Treatment

- Can give vitamin A, antivirals (eg, ribavirin) and human immunoglobulin (Ig)
  - *Give at 6 mos. MMR Vaccine to pediatric patients*

Conjunctivitis

Definition

- Any inflammation of the sclera due to bacterial or viral infection

Bilateral: Infectious or allergic.
Unilateral: Toxic, chemical, mechanical, or lacrimal in origin

Clinical Presentation

- Patient has inflamed conjunctiva with severe photophobia and foreign-body sensation

Treatment

- Cefotaxime or besifloxacin (4th gen Fluoroquinolone)
- **Bacterial**: Make sure to cover for MRSA
- **Viral:** Supportive

Down Syndrome

Definition

- MC chromosomal disorder in humans and the MC cause of intellectual disability. It is primarily caused by *trisomy of chromosome 21*

Clinical Presentation

- Flat occiput and a flattened facial appearance, Epicanthal folds, flat nasal bridge
- Upward-slanting palpebral fissures, *Brushfield spots*, Protruding tongue, Small and dysplastic ears, Single transverse palmar crease (simian), Short fifth finger with clinodactyly and commonly a wide space between the first and second toes

Cystic Fibrosis

Definition

- Disease of *exocrine gland dysfunction* that involves multiple organ systems but results in chronic respiratory infections, pancreatic enzyme insufficiency, and associated complications in untreated patients
- CF males have 75 to 80% with *congenital bilateral absence of vas deferens*

MC mutation. *Delta F508 gene* on chromosome 7
Gold standard diagnosis: *Sweat chloride test* (>60 mEq/L) and

Treatment

- Pancreatic enzyme supplements
- Multivitamins (including fat-soluble vitamins)
- Mucolytics
- Nebulized, inhaled, oral, or intravenous antibiotics
- Bronchodilators
- Anti-inflammatory agents
- Agents to treat associated conditions or complications (insulin, bisphosphonates)

Turner Syndrome

Definition

- One of the MC chromosomal abnormalities, occurring in approximately 1 in 2000 live-born *female infants*

- Turner syndrome is caused by the absence of one set of genes from the short arm of one X chromosome

Clinical Workup

- Confirmed by the *presence of a 45,X cell line* or a cell line with deletion of the short arm of the X chromosome (Xp deletion)
- The buccal smear for Barr bodies is obsolete
    - A *male phenotype excludes the diagnosis*, regardless of karyotype

Signs

- 95% have *short stature* and *signs of ovarian failure* upon physical examination

Short stature: Before age 11 years, height and growth are well within the normal range, but heights are below the 50th percentile for girls with Turners.

Dental: A high arched palate

Ovarian failure

- No breast development by age 12 years or have not started menses by age 14 years
- Elevated levels of luteinizing hormone (LH) and FSH confirm ovarian failure

Nevi: Excessive numbers of nevi. These may be removed if rubbed or irritated by clothing

Webbed neck: Lymphedema in utero can cause a broad neck and a low or indistinct hairline

Chapter Five

Geriatrics

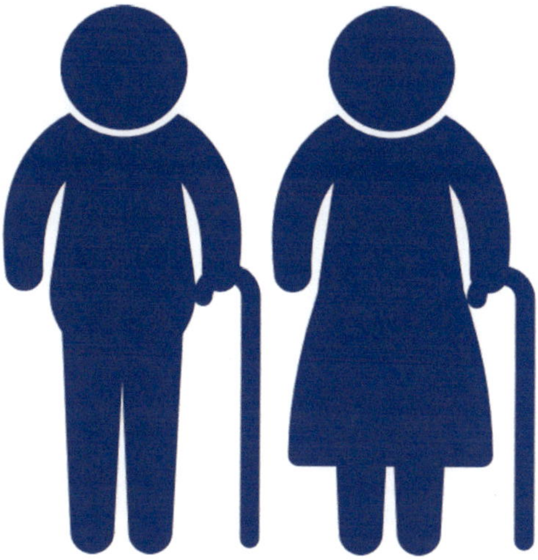

Shingles

Definition

- An acute, cutaneous viral infection caused by the *reactivation of varicella-zoster virus* (VZV)

Clinical Presentation

Prodrome: An interval of pain prior to onset of cutaneous findings

- Patchy erythema, fever and local lymphadenopathy
- *Grouped herpetiform vesicles developing on the erythematous base,* Generally follows a dermatome pattern

If patient develops *pain in pre-auricular area that radiates to the eye* and patient has a *vesicle on nose*: Refer to ophthalmologist immediately: (Herpes Zoster) causing optic neuritis.

Labs

- The Tzanck smear confirms that the lesion is herpetic *but cannot differentiate* between VZV and other herpes viruses

Treatment

- Acyclovir and its derivatives (*Famciclovir, penciclovir, and valacyclovir*) have been shown to be safe and effective in the treatment of active disease and the prevention of postherpetic neuralgia (PHN)

Renal Cell Carcinoma

Definition

- This is the *most common type of kidney cancer in adults* and accounts for 90-95% of renal tumors
- 25-30% have metastatic disease at diagnosis
- 5% have a solitary metastasis

Clinical Presentation

Classic triad (10%): *Hematuria, flank pain and palpable abdominal mass*

- Others: Fever, weight loss, HTN, night sweats, malaise

Labs

- UA, CBC, LFT/ AST/ ALT

Imaging

- PET scan, *CT scan*, MRI

Treatment

- 50% cure rate: Surgery, Chemotherapy, and Rad therapy

Renal cell carcinoma is an immunogenic tumor and there are many spontaneous regressions. (INF, IL-2 has also been tried with some success)

ACE Inhibitors

Definition

- ACE (Angiotensin Converting Enzyme) inhibitors; inhibit the activity of the enzyme ACE that decreases the production of angiotensin II

Clinical Presentation

- Patient generally presents with HTN (*>140/80*) and has failed lifestyle modifications
- Ace Inhibitors (*Ramapril, Captopril, Benazapril, Enalapril, Fosinopril, Lisinopril*)

Treatment Indications

- ACE inhibitors have been proven to decrease mortality and morbidity
- Before a patient is discharged from the hospital after having an MI, he must be put on an ACE inhibitor
- The ACE Inhibitor may need renal dosing and is *renal protective for those with HTN and DM* who do not have previous renal disease as this is (*first line treatment*)

Alzheimer's

Definition

- Alzheimer's is an acquired disorder of cognitive and behavioral impairment that markedly interferes with social and occupational functioning
- It is a *long, progressive incurable disease*

Physiology

- *Amyloid precursor protein (APP)* breaks at the B-subunit and B-amyloid plaques develop that have reactive halos what deposit in certain regions of the brain that is associated with memory

Risk Factors

- The greatest known risk factor for Alzheimer's is *advancing age*
- Most individuals with the disease are age 65 or older
- The likelihood of developing Alzheimer's disease doubles *every five years after the age of 65*
- After age 85, the risk reaches nearly 50 percent

Imaging

- CT scan and PET scan exclude other possible causes for dementia (cerebrovascular disease, cobalamin [*vitamin B12*] deficiency, syphilis, thyroid disease)

Clinical Presentation

- Specific regions of the brain (Entorhinal cortex and hippocampus) begin to be affected *10-20 years before any visible symptoms* appear
- B-Amyloid plaques may develop as early as the 5th decade

Treatment

- Only symptomatic therapy is available to date
- These medications MC include: Antidepressants, Anxiolytics, Anti-parkinsonian agents, Beta-blockers, Antiepileptic drugs (for their effects on behavior) and Neuroleptics

Age Related Macular Degeneration (ARMD)

Definition

- This is the *most common cause of irreversible vision loss* among the elderly
- ARMD is caused by a pathologic choroidal neovascular membrane (CNVM) that develops under the retina and can leak fluid and blood

Clinical Presentation

- This is often asymptomatic or have mild symptoms, including *minimally blurred central visual acuity*, contrast and color disturbances

Exudative (Wet)

- *Painless progressive blurring* of their central visual acuity, which can be acute or insidious in onset

Non-Exudative (Dry)

- *90% of patients diagnosed with ARMD*
- Associated with the *presence of drusen*, without visual loss early in the disease, and often progresses to retinal atrophy and central retinal degeneration with associated loss of central vision. *Takes decades to develop.*

Treatment

Exudative

- Ranibizumab: An intra-vitreally injected, recombinant, humanized, monoclonal antibody fragment designed to *actively bind and inhibit all isoforms of VEGF*

Non-Exudative

- *No medical treatment*: Recommended to consume adequate quantities of antioxidants, including vitamin A, vitamin E, zinc, and lutein

Activities of Daily Living (ADL)

Definition

- Tasks that are required to get going in the morning, get from place to place using one's body, and then close out the day in the evening. They involve caring for and moving the body

Include: Walking, bathing, dressing, toileting, brushing teeth, eating

Instrumental Activities of daily Living (IADLs)

Definition

- Activities that people do once they are up, dressed, put together. These tasks support an independent life style. Many people can still live independently even though they need help with one or two of these IADL's

Include: Cooking, driving, using the telephone or computer, shopping, keeping track of finances, and managing medication

Osteoporosis

Definition

- This is the *most common metabolic bone disease in the United States* and can result in devastating physical, psychosocial, and economic consequences

Risk Factors

- White female, >55yo, Fracture in a first degree relative, smoking, estrogen deficiency, Low calcium intake, alcoholism and low amounts of physical exercise

Clinical Presentation

- Patients are often overweight and have multiple risk factors. They are generally female and over 55 years old (however, this can occur in men)

Imaging

- Dual-energy X-ray Absorptiometry (*DXA*) and bone mineral density (BMD)

Treatment

- *Bisphosphonates*, Selective Estrogen-Receptor Modulator (SERM) raloxifene, calcitonin, and denosumab
- All therapy should be given with calcium and vitamin D

T-score/Z-score for Osteoporosis/Guidelines

T score: Compared to 30-year-old bones

Z score: Age adjusted comparing 70 year old bones to the average DEXA scan of all 70 year old olds

DEXA scan *every 1-2 years for men and women >65 yo*

Some of the risk factors

- History of bone fracture as an adult
- Current smoking
- History of ever taking oral steroids for more than 3 months
- Body weight under 127 pounds
- Having an immediate family member with a fragility fracture (a broken bone from a minor injury, suggesting osteoporosis)

Definition (Bone Mass)	Bone Mass Density	T-Score
Normal	W/in 1 SD of Mean bone density for young women	$\geq$ -1
Low (Osteopenia)	1-2.5 SD below the mean	-1 and -2.5
Osteoporosis	$\geq$ 2.5 *SSSS* below the normal mean	$\leq$ -2.5
Severe Osteoporosis	$\geq$ 2.5 *SSSS* below the normal mean for young- adult with > 1 fracture	$\leq$ -2.5 with fracture

Tardive Dyskinesia

Definition

- It is *involuntary movements of the tongue, lips, face, trunk, and extremities* that occur in patients treated with long-term dopaminergic antagonist medications

Causes

- MC chronic treatment of cholinesterase inhibitors causes what (donepezil, rivastigmine)

Treatment

- Atypical antipsychotics, such as Risperidone and clozapine, appear to have a lower risk of tardive dyskinesia
- Always use the lowest effective dose for the shortest possible period

Vaccines for Elderly

It is recommended that elderly persons *over the age of 65* should receive

- Influenza (Flu) -*Yearly*
- Shingles (Herpes Zoster)
- Diphtheria
- Tetanus
- Pertussis (Whooping Cough)
- Pneumococcal disease (Pneumonia)

Nursing Home Placement

Causes

- *Dementia is the #1 cause of Skilled Nursing placement*. Dementia patients are often too overwhelming (mentally and physically) for family caregivers and can lead to increased rates of elderly abuse and neglect

Anticholinergic Drugs

Relevance

- Could *increase the risk for Dementia* (Dose response) Tricyclic antidepressants and oxybutynin were the closest linked. Also linked to ataxia. *Contraindicated in people with mental status changes*

Treatment

- *Do not use in patients with mental status changes* as blocking the synthesis of acetylcholine in a patient that is already insufficient can make the patient's condition worse
  - Oxybutynin- over active bladder
  - Tricyclic Antidepressants

Pressure Ulcers

Definition

- This is an area of unrelieved pressure over a defined area, usually over a bony prominence, resulting in ischemia, cell death, and tissue necrosis

Stage 1	Intact skin with non-blanchable redness in a localized area
Stage 2	Partial thickness loss of dermis
Stage 3	Full Thickness loss of tissue. SubQ fat may be seen.
Stage 4	Full Thickness with exposed tendon, muscle or bone

Clinical Presentation

- *First sign of ulcer is unblanchable skin*, localized redness usually over boney or darkly pigmented skin

Labs

Albumin

- A **low albumin** level (less that 3.5 g/dl) is indicative of several potential problems including: *cirrhosis, malnutrition, or kidney disease*
- Also linked to an increase in mortality and is a sign of poor healing and dehydration

Treatment/ Education

- The key to successful management is reduction of pressure, adequate debridement of necrotic and devitalized tissue, Control of infection and meticulous wound care

Benign Prostatic Hypertrophy

Definition

- This is a histologic diagnosis characterized by proliferation of the cellular elements of the prostate

Clinical Presentation

- Patients often presents with (*Chronic Bladder Outlet Obstruction*), secondarily causing urinary retention, renal insufficiency, recurrent urinary tract infections, gross hematuria, and bladder calculi
- Patients are generally at least *55 years old* but may present sooner

Treatment

- Transurethral resection of the prostate (*TURP*) is the *gold standard* for relieving bladder outlet obstruction in patients with BPH
- *Alpha-adrenergic receptor–blocking agents* an also be administered and act by decreasing resistance along the bladder neck, prostate, and urethra by relaxing the smooth muscle and allowing passage of urine

Cautions

- *If patient is on any kind of nitrate, avoid (PDE 5 inhibitors)*
- PDE-5 inhibitors prevent the breakdown of nitrates and causes prolonged vasodilation, which could plummet BP and cause cerebral and myocardial hypo profusion
- Sildenafil (Viagra) or Nitro tabs: MC

Incontinence

Definition

- This is the involuntary loss of urine that represents a hygienic or social problem to the individual

Clinical Presentation

- This affects about 50-84% of the elderly in long-term care facilities and it is most common among women

Types

Stress	Urine leakage associated with increased abdominal pressure from laughing, sneezing, coughing, climbing stairs, or other physical stressors on the abdominal cavity and the bladder
Urge	Involuntary leakage accompanied by or immediately preceded by urgency
Mixed	A combination of stress and urge incontinence, marked by involuntary leakage associated with urgency and also with exertion, effort, sneezing, or coughing
Functional	The inability to hold urine due to reasons other than neuro-urologic and lower urinary tract dysfunction (delirium, psychiatric disorders, urinary infection, impaired mobility)

Treatment

- First line therapy for stress incontinence is *pelvic floor exercises*.
- Patients in skilled nursing facilities should have *timed restroom breaks Q2 hrs*
- Medical treatment includes Oxybutynin, however *this is contraindicated* if the patient has ataxia, confusion or any signs of mental status change

CAM Criteria

Definition

This is (Confusion Assessment Method), which is the *criteria to diagnose delirium*

The Test

Part 1: An assessment instrument that screens for *overall cognitive impairment*

Part 2: Includes only *four features* that were found to have the greatest ability to distinguish delirium or reversible confusion from other types of cognitive impairment

- **Feature 1:** Acute Onset and Fluctuating Course
- **Feature 2:** Inattention
- **Feature 3:** Disorganized thinking
- **Feature 4:** Altered Level of consciousness

Lumbar Radiculopathies

Definition

- Radiculopathy is a result of nerve root impingement, disc herniation and facet arthropathy
- This is *not a cause of low back pain*

Clinical Presentation

- Patients can present with *burning, shooting pain, numbness and tingling* generally in a nerve root distribution associated with their symptoms. If an elderly person has weakness in the lower extremity use a:
  - Walker- for support
  - If there is no weakness but just ataxia, use a cane for balance

Treatment

First Line

- (*Excluding Cauda Equine Syndrome*) Core strengthening, Spine traction, Epidural steroid injection and Nerve blocks

Surgical options

- Simple discectomy, Discectomy plus fusion, Chemo-nucleosis, Percutaneous discectomy and Micro-discectomy

Imaging

- **Plain films** are not necessary for most episodes of acute LBP, especially *within the first 6 weeks* after the onset of symptoms

- **MRI** has excellent sensitivity in the diagnosis of lumbar disc herniation and is considered the *imaging study of choice* for nerve root impingement

Lewy Body Dementia

Definition

- This is a progressive, degenerative dementia of unknown etiology

Clinical Presentation

- *Visual hallucinations and agitation*
- Fluctuating cognition with pronounced variations in attention and alertness
- Recurrent complex visual hallucinations, typically well-formed and detailed
- Spontaneous features of Parkinsonism
- Can have personality changes

Histology

- The characteristic lesion is the LB, an *eosinophilic (hematoxylin and eosin staining), round inclusion* found in the cytoplasm of substantia nigra cells

Labs

- CSF levels of beta amyloid are lower than normal
- SPECT or positron emission tomography (PET) scanning shows decreased occipital lobe blood flow or metabolism, which is not seen in Alzheimer disease

Treatment

- Cholinesterase Inhibitors such as (Donepezil, Rivastigmine) can increase acetylcholine
- Symptomatic relief of agitation, sleeplessness and hallucinations

Elderly Screening Guidelines

- Chest X-ray- (if no cardio risk)
- Medicare covers colorectal screening every 12 mo.
- Pneumonia vaccine yearly
- Lipid panel Q 5 yrs. or yearly if significant risk factors
- All patients with AAA or Hx of AAA or *smoked 100 cigarettes* can screen with *abdominal aneurism*. Must be between 65-75 years old

Ophthalmic Exam Recommendation

Recommendation is every 1-2 years

- A person may need more frequent exams (perhaps even more often than once a year) if he has certain medical conditions, like diabetes or high blood pressure, which may put him at higher risk for some eye diseases

There should be an *ophthalmologist consult* if the patient

- Takes certain medications
- Has had a serious eye injury in the past
- Is African American (because of the increased risk of glaucoma)
- Has a personal or family history of eye disease

Parkinson's

Definition

- This is one of the *most common neurologic disorders*, affecting approximately 1% of individuals older than 60 years and causing progressive disability that can be slowed, but not stopped by treatment

Clinical Presentation

- "*Rolling pill tremor*"
- Often have depression, masked faces, constipation and forgetfulness

- **Two Features**
  - *Loss of pigmented dopaminergic neurons* of the substantia nigra pars compacta
  - *The presence of Lewy bodies* and Lewy neuritis
- **4 Cardinal Signs**
  - Resting tremor, Rigidity, Bradykinesia, Postural instability

Treatment

- *Gold standard is to replace the dopamine* that is no longer being made
- Carbidopa/Levodopa (Sinemet, Amantadine or Apomorphine) are the main medications
  - Side effects (orthostatic hypotension)

Amurosis Feagoux

Definition

- This is a *transient visual loss* and is a frequently encountered complaint that, in most cases, has an identifiable cause. If it is associated with a TIA, it will last *< 24 hours*. It is most commonly due to a transient ischemic event.

Imaging

- U/S carotids: must rule out Trans Ischemic Attach (TIA)

Treatment

- This is dependent on the cause. An investigation of any cardiovascular and cerebrovascular events should take place.

Get Up and Go Test

Definition

- Very simple and sensitive screen for (Activities of Daily Living)

Test Procedure

- Start sitting in a chair
- Stand without using hands to push upwards

- Walk 10 feet
- Turn around and walk back to the chair
- Sit down

Normal Results: <10 seconds
Impaired Results: >20 seconds

Hospice

- Do not accept people looking for palliative or curative care
- Patients are expected to *have <6 months to live*
- Hospice provides Comfort care, which is an essential part of medical **care** at the end of life. It is **care** that helps or soothes a person who is dying. The goal is to prevent or relieve suffering as much as possible while respecting the dying person's wishes.
- *Palliative care*: The goal is to improve quality of life for both the patient and the family

Bereavement

Definition

- The grieving process is *natural* and unique to each individual and shares some of the same features of depression such as *intense sadness* and *withdrawal from customary activities*

Differences between Grief and Depression	
Grief	**Depression**
Painful feelings come in waves, often intermixed with positive memories of the deceased	Mood and ideation are almost constantly negative
Self-esteem is usually preserved	Corrosive feelings of worthlessness and self-loathing are common
Depression *should not be diagnosed* in the context of bereavement since the diagnosis would *incorrectly label a normal process as a disorder*	

Pneumonia

Definition

- PNA is a clinical diagnosis what has segmental or lobar distribution of infiltrates in CXR and can have vascular markings that suggest volume overload CHF

Clinical Presentation

- MC Fever, cough, chest pain, or rapid respiration. Patients with COPD and Chronic Bronchitis are most susceptible.
- *PNA is the #1 cause of infectious death in the elderly*.
- Significant cause of mortality and morbidity among residents of such facilities

Community Acquired Pneumonia

- (MC pathogens): *Streptococcus pneumonia, Haemophilus influenza, Moraxella catarrhalis*

Treatment

- Antibiotic therapy specific to the organism being targeted should be initiated
- Aspergillus and viral PNA does not respond to antibiotics

Temporal Arteritis

Definition

- This is an inflammatory reaction involving the *temporal artery* and other *medium-sized arteries* of the head & neck

Clinical Presentation

- Visual disturbances, headache, jaw claudication, neck pain, and scalp tenderness. Constitutional manifestations, such as fatigue, malaise, and fever, may also be present

Labs: Increased ESR

Treatment

Tx with high dose methylprednisolone

- Damage may be irreversible after 48 hrs
- The major justification for the use of corticosteroids is the impending danger of blindness in untreated patients

Major Depression

Definition (DSM-5)

- Must have *at least 5 symptoms* that must have been presented *during the same 2-week period* (and at least 1 of the symptoms must be diminished interest/pleasure or depressed mood)
- Anhedonia, insomnia, psychomotor agitation, fatigue, feelings of worthlessness, can't concentrate and recurrent thoughts of death

Clinical Presentation

- Presenting complaints are mostly somatic, such as fatigue, headache, abdominal distress, or sleep problems

Treatment

First line: (Celexa, Citalopram or Sertraline)

- SSRIs are considered to have the *best safety profile in the elderly* because they have the lowest potential for drug-drug in-teractions based on their cyto-chrome P-450 interactions
- The *SSRI Fluoxetine is not recommended* in the elderly because of the increased half-life of the drug

Dehydration

Definition

- This is a state of negative fluid balance that may be caused by numerous disease entities
- This is very common in elderly on diuretics

Clinical Presentation

- Increased heart rate, increased thirst, dry mouth, weakness, dizziness, palpitations (feeling that the heart is jumping or pounding), confusion, sluggishness, fainting, inability to sweat, decreased urine output

Treatment

- Oral rehydration for mild or moderate dehydration unless the patient is vomiting
- Severe dehydration: Intravenous rapid administration of 20 mL/kg of an isotonic crystalloid (lactated Ringer solution, 0.9% sodium chloride)

Candidiasis

Definition

- This is a fungal infection caused by yeasts from the genus Candida

Clinical presentation

- Most commonly present with disfiguring lesions of the face, scalp, hands, and nails. Chronic mucocutaneous candidiasis is occasionally associated with oral thrush and vitiligo

Oropharyngeal candidiasis (OPC) usually have a *history of HIV infection*, wear dentures, have diabetes mellitus, exposed to broad-spectrum antibiotics or inhaled steroids. This looks like a curdy appearance in the back of the throat.

Treatment

- Azoles such as fluconazole are the mainstay therapy for Candidiasis

Elderly falls

- Illnesses and physical conditions can affect your *strength and balance*
- Normal changes of aging, like *poor eyesight* or *poor hearing*, can make you more likely to fall
- *Poor lighting* or throw rugs in your home can make you more likely to trip or slip
- The *side effects of some medicines* can upset your balance and make you fall
    - Anti-depressives and hypertension medications often cause falls. Some medicines for diabetes and heart conditions can also cause ataxia.

Beers List

This is a long list of Medications that should be avoided in the elderly with certain conditions.

Chapter Six

Emergency Medicine

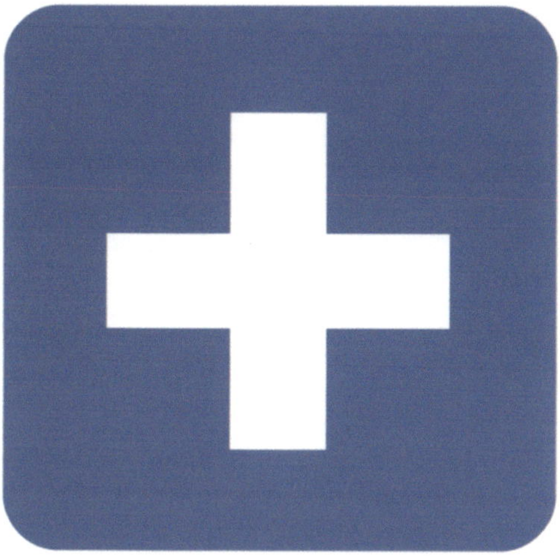

Epiglottitis

Definition

- An Acute inflammatory condition of the epiglottis that may progress rapidly to a life threatening airway obstruction

Clinical presentation

Children

- Abrupt onset of high fever, sore throat, dysphagia (difficulty swallowing), muffled voice, drooling, and stridor. Usually appear toxic and anxious. Rare d/t Hib Vaccinations.

Adults

- Often present with a several day prodrome of *upper respiratory tract infection* and a severe sore throat that is out of proportion to clinical findings

Diagnostic Evaluation

- Plain film imaging of the lateral neck: swollen epiglottis ("**Thumbprint Sign**")
- Stridor, voice muffling, rapid clinical course, and a history of diabetes mellitus are associated with the need for airway intervention
    - Sore throat~95%
    - Odynophagia/dysphagia (95%)
    - Muffled voice (54%) - "Hot potato voice"

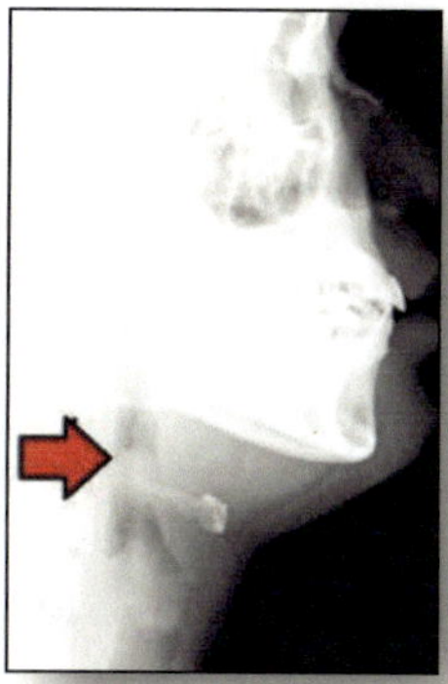

Figure 5: By Med Chaos (Own work) [CC0], via Wikimedia Commons

Treatment

- Ensure a patent airway (intubation), oxygen, IV fluids, IV antibiotics (ceftriaxone), and steroids. May also give anti pyretic (ASA, Tylenol)
- Consultation with ENT

Subarachnoid Hemorrhage

Definition

- Extravasation of blood into the subarachnoid space between the pial and arachnoid membranes

Risk Factors

- HTN, smoking, cocaine use, prior SAH, family history of SAH.
- Associated with polycystic kidney dz.

Cause

- Disruption of the parenchyma and subarachnoid vessels
- MC d/t trauma
- Also caused by ruptured saccular aneurysms usually within or near the circle of Willis, or an AV malformation

Clinical presentation

- Sudden, severe headache. "**Worst headache of my life**" "**Thunderclap headache**"
- Neck and back pain may be present due to dural inflammation extending down the spine

Diagnosis

- Non-contrast head CT with or without lumbar puncture
- A negative head CT and lumbar puncture effectively eliminates the diagnosis of SAH as long as both tests are performed
- Sensitivity of head CT for detecting SAH is highest in first 6 to 12 hours
- Best to follow-up with a lumbar puncture when a CT scan is negative

Clearing of blood in progressive tubes of LP

- Traumatic LP --- not SAH

Xanthrochromia

- Pink or yellow tint of CSF that represents hemoglobin degradation products
- LP is most accurate after 12 hours of symptoms when Xanthrochromia may be present

Treatment

- Antihypertensive agents when the mean arterial pressure *(MAP) exceeds 130 mm Hg*
- Intravenous beta-blockers, have a relatively short half-life, can be titrated easily and do not increase intracranial pressure (ICP)
- *Beta-blockers are the agents of choice in patients without contraindications*
- *Avoid nitrates* such as nitroprusside or nitroglycerin, which elevate ICP

Types of Headaches

Time of Onset

- Chronic headache (duration of months or more) is usually not due to a serious disorder
- Headache of acute onset or of a changing pain pattern demands prompt evaluation
- Determine if the headache differs from or is identical to the patient's chronic problem
- Headaches in the early morning or those causing waking may indicate an increase in ICP and evaluation for intracranial tumor

Family History of Headaches

- Primary headache disorders have a family history of headaches

4 types of primary headaches

Tension-type

- Tight, *band-like*, NOT throbbing. Improves with activity. Mild to moderate in intensity.
- *Bilateral* and lasts hours to days, no N/V. May be light or sound sensitivity, but not both. Stress, fatigue, lack or sleep, Hx of depression/anxiety is triggers
- Caused by continuous contraction of head and neck muscles, possibly triggered by stress

Cluster headache: **usually unilateral and cyclic**

- *Autonomic phenomena*: Ptosis, miosis (constriction of pupil), lacrimation, and rhinorrhea/nasal congestion
- Lasts 15 min to 2-3 hours, can get *multiple in a day*. "*Boring*" or "*stabbing*" pain
- Location of pain: *behind or above the eye or in temple*, but can also be check, teeth, jaw, or forehead
- Triggers: alcohol, nitroglycerin and histamine
- No GI upset or light sensitivity
- Occur in groups over weeks/months, then not occur at all for weeks-months

Migraine headache

- Lasts hours to days. *Unilateral* usually. Throbbing, worse with activity.
- Nausea and/or vomiting. Photophobia and phonophobia (sound sensitivity). May have an aura. Cutaneous allodynia-skin hurts to the touch.
- Can have prodrome 1-2 days before attack, and aura 1-2 hours before attack (Aura: Transient episodes of focal neurologic dysfunction, dizziness, unilateral numbness or weakness, anxiety, hyperventilation, dysphagia)
- Other: Exertional, cough headache, etc.

Location of Pain

Migraine or the Cluster Variant	Hemicranial (*unilateral*) or retroocular pain
Tension Headache	Commonly diffuse, occipital, or *bandlike* pain
Mass Lesion Headache	Often-focal "*right here*"
Trigeminal Neuralgia	Stabbing pain localized to the second or third division of the trigeminal nerve

Quality of Pain

Migraine or the Cluster Variant	Commonly described as throbbing and often preceded by prodromal symptoms or auras, for example, scintillating scotoma or other visual changes
Tension Headache and Mass Lesion Headache	Usually steady pain
Trigeminal Neuralgia	Shooting or stabbing character

Timing

Mass Lesion Headache

- *Worst when awakening*

Cluster Variant of Migraine

- Frequently awaken patients from sleep and often recur at the same time of day or night

Tension Headache

- May develop at regular intervals, especially with recurrent stressful situations

Factors Influencing Severity

Migraine of the Cluster Variant

- Frequently relieved by pressure on the ipsilateral temporal or carotid artery; by darkness, sleep, or vomiting; or during pregnancy

Mass Lesion Headache

- Often exacerbated by events such as coughing and sneezing that transiently raise intracranial pressure. Valsalva maneuver

Precipitating Factors

Tension Headache

- Tension, emotional stress, and fatigue

Migraine

- Hunger, nitrite-containing foods (hot dogs, salami, sausage), chocolate, aged cheeses, bright lights, menses, alcohol, caffeine, monosodium glutamate, aspartame, and insomnia

Cluster Variant of Migraine

- Alcohol

Trigeminal Neuralgia and the Jaw Claudication of Temporal Arteritis

- Chewing and eating

Associated Symptoms

- *Nausea or vomiting* is common with migraine and may be seen late in the course of mass lesions
- *Photophobia* is prominent with migraine headache but occurs also with meningitis, especially viral (aseptic) meningitis
- *Myalgias* of pericranial muscles (posterior neck muscles) often accompany tension headaches and viral syndromes

- *Rhinorrhea* and lacrimation during headache typify the cluster variant of migraine and are ipsilateral to the pain

Temporal Arteritis (Giant Cell Arteritis)

- Form of vasculitis that may cause a HA
- (MC) Autoimmune in origin
- Typically affect the elderly, 4X as common in women; complain of sharp, burning, unilateral pain that may be worse at night

Physical Exam

- Tender pulseless superficial temporal artery, decreased visual acuity
- ESR (non-specific marker of inflammation) will be elevated

Can cause blindness: Immediate treatment with steroids to reduce inflammation is warranted.

Treatment of headaches

- *NSAIDS*: best for *tension headaches*
- *Oxygen therapy*: *cluster headaches*
- Ergots: Ergotamine, DHE (dihydroergotamine)→these are vasoconstrictors
- Anti-emetics
- Triptans

GI bleeding

- **Duodenal Ulcer**- Pain relieved by eating
- **Stomach Ulcer**- Pain made worse with eating
- **GI bleeds:** gastric ulcer: coffee ground emesis

Asthma

Definition

- Variable airflow limitation and airway hyper-responsiveness
- Airway inflammation
- Recurrent airway obstruction that is *reversible*

Atopy

- Genetic predisposition to develop IgE antibodies directed against common environmental allergens is the *strongest identifiable risk factor* for asthma development

Clinical presentation

- Episodes of wheezing, breathlessness, chest tightness, and coughing, particularly at night or in the early morning

Treatment

- Adrenergic agonists (Albuterol) are the preferred initial rescue medication for acute bronchospasm
- Corticosteroids are highly effective drugs in asthma exacerbation
- ***Methacholine challenge:*** (bronchoconstriction)
- **Drop is FEV1/FVC greater than 20%** observed: Asthma

Pulmonary Embolism

Definition

- A blood clot that arises from thrombi that originates in the deep venous system of the lower extremities
- 90% come from lower extremities as a DVT

Risk Factors

- Recent travel
- Surgery within last 3 months
- Malignancy
- Smoking
- Hx of thrombophlebitis
- Prior PE, Heart Failure or COPD

Clinical Presentation

- MC: Abrupt onset of pleuritic chest pain, shortness of breath, and hypoxia

Key Words: "*Wedge shape on x-ray for PE → Westermark sign*"

Treatment

- Low-molecular weight heparin (LMWH) or fondaparinux
- Thrombolytic therapy for: Acute PE associated with hypotension (*Systolic BP < 90 mm Hg*)

Anterior Nose Bleed with Known Source

First line

Basic tamponade maneuvers

- Patient blows their nose to remove blood and clots
- Clinician sprays the nose with oxymetazoline (**Afrin**) to hasten hemostasis through vasoconstriction
- Patient **pinches the anterior aspect** of nose tightly against the septum and holds continuously for ten minutes
- **Head position forward** is preferred so no blood is aspirated or swallowed
- Most episodes will resolve with *simple direct pressure*

Second line

Chemical cautery: Silver nitrate

Electrical cautery

- Both can cause rhinorrhea, crusting, ulceration, perforation
- Never done bilaterally due to risk of sepal necrosis

Third line

Nasal tampons

- Topical anesthetic and vasoconstrictor, coat in Bactrim (Avoid toxic-shock syndrome), insert and infuse tampon with 10mL of saline to inflate

Gauze packing

- Ribbon gauze impregnated with petroleum

Balloon catheters

- Topical anesthetic and vasoconstrictor, soak in sterile water, until fabric ring reaches the nares and then inflate the balloon with air

ECG Highlights

This section was made possible with permission of use from Dr. Mike Tadogan MD, an emergency physician in Australia. Check out his blog for the best comprehensive review of ECG's. The following ECG strips are some of the most common seen in practice and on exams.

http://lifeinthefastlane.com/ecg-library/

Ventricular Tachycardia

- Broad complex tachycardia originating in the ventricles
- There are several different varieties of VT: MC type is Monomorphic VT

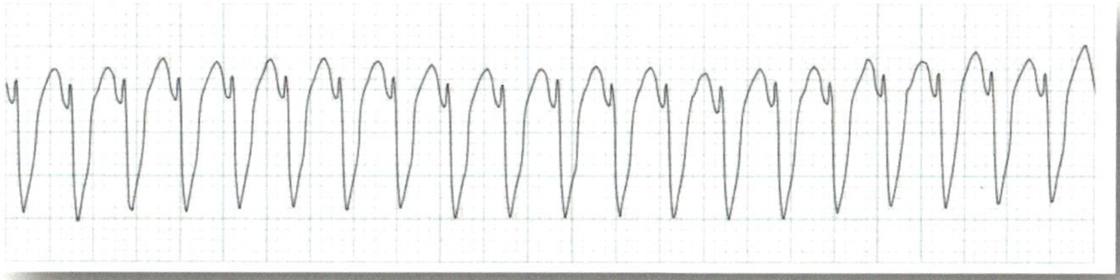

Clinical Significance

- Ventricular tachycardia may impair cardiac output with consequent hypotension, collapse, and acute cardiac failure. This is due to *extreme heart rates* and lack of coordinated atrial contraction (*loss of "atrial kick"*)
- The presence of pre-existing poor ventricular function is strongly associated with cardiovascular compromise
- Decreased cardiac output may result in decreased myocardial perfusion with *degeneration to VF*
- Prompt recognition and initiation of treatment (*electrical cardioversion*) is required in all cases of VT

Ventricular Fibrillation

Findings

- Chaotic irregular deflections of varying amplitude
- No identifiable P waves, QRS complexes, or T waves
- Rate *150 to 500* per minute
- Amplitude decreases with duration (coarse VF -> fine VF)

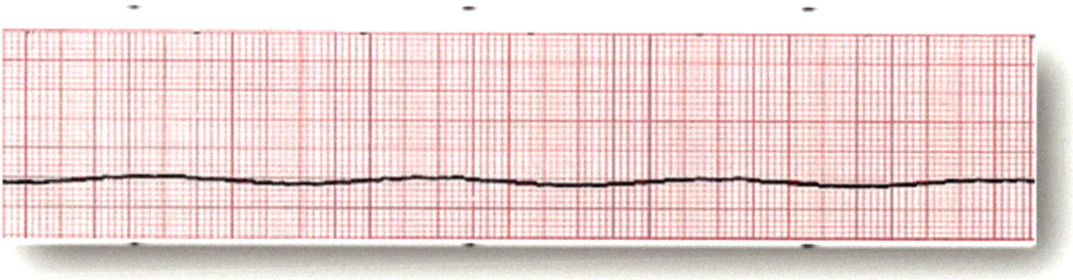

Clinical Significance

- Must *cardiovert* patient or this rhythm is fatal

Asystole

Definition

- No cardiac electrical activity, hence *no contractions of the myocardium* and no cardiac output or blood flow

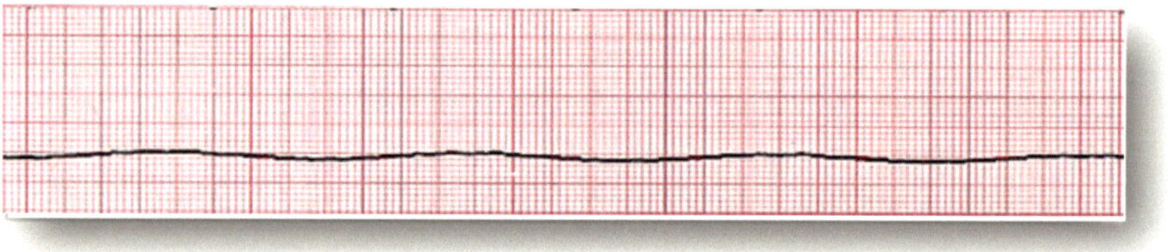

Clinical Significance: Must *cardiovert* or rhythm is fatal.
Atrial flutter:

Sinus Tachycardia

Definition

- Sinus rhythm with a resting *heart rate of > 100 bpm* in adults, or above the normal range for age in children
- **Newborn**: 110 – 150 bpm
- **2 years**: 85 – 125 bpm
- **4 years**: 75 – 115 bpm
- **6 years+**: 60 – 100 bpm

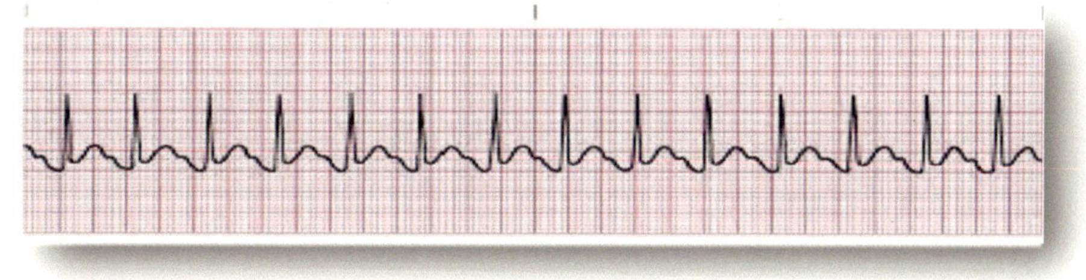

Sinus Bradycardia

Definition

- When the heart rate is <60 bpm
- Common to find prominent "U" waves in the precordial leads

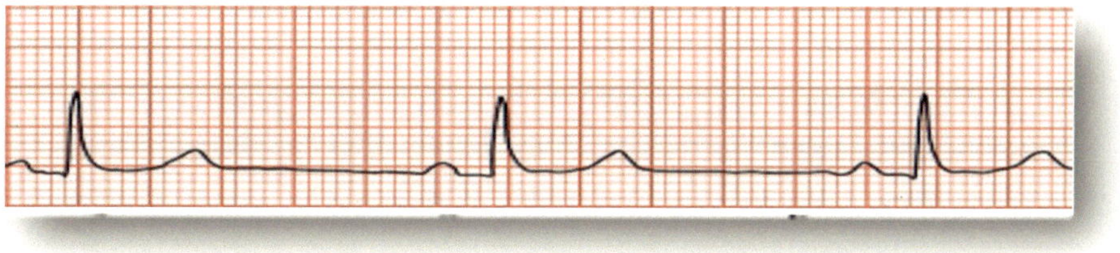

Clinical Significance

- If the HR gets to low you can experience syncope or organ failure.
- Newborn: 110 – 150 bpm
- 2 years: 85 – 125 bpm
- 4 years: 75 – 115 bpm
- 6 years+: 60 – 100 bpm

AV Heart Blocks

First Degree

Definition

- PR interval > 200ms (five small squares)
- ‘Marked’ first degree block if PR interval > 300ms

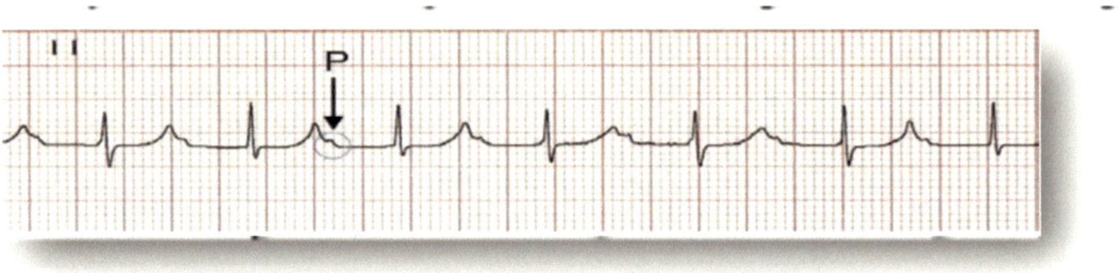

Clinical Significance

- Does not cause hemodynamic disturbance
- No specific treatment is required

Second Degree

Mobitz I (Wenchebach)

Definition

- Progressive *prolongation of the PR* interval culminating in a *non-conducted P wave*
- The PR interval is *longest* immediately before the dropped beat
- The PR interval is *shortest* immediately after the dropped beat

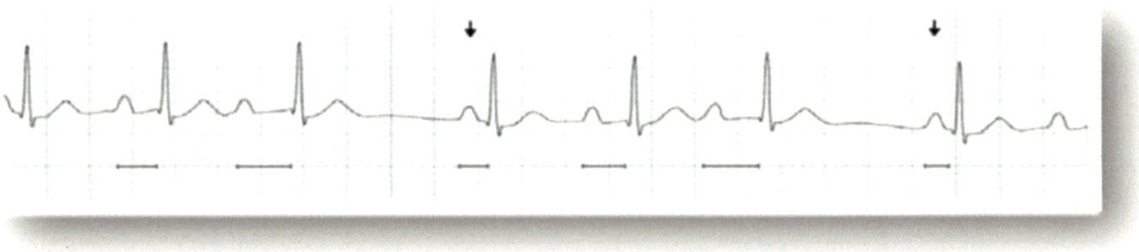

Clinical Significance

- Mobitz I is usually a *benign rhythm*, causing *minimal hemodynamic disturbance* and with low risk of progression to third degree heart block

- Asymptomatic patients do *not require treatment*
- Symptomatic patients usually respond to *atropine*

Mobitz II

Definition

- Intermittent non-conducted P waves without progressive prolongation of the PR interval
- The *PR interval* in the conducted beats *remains constant*.
- The *P waves 'march through'* at a constant rate
- The RR interval surrounding the dropped beat(s) is an exact multiple of the preceding RR interval

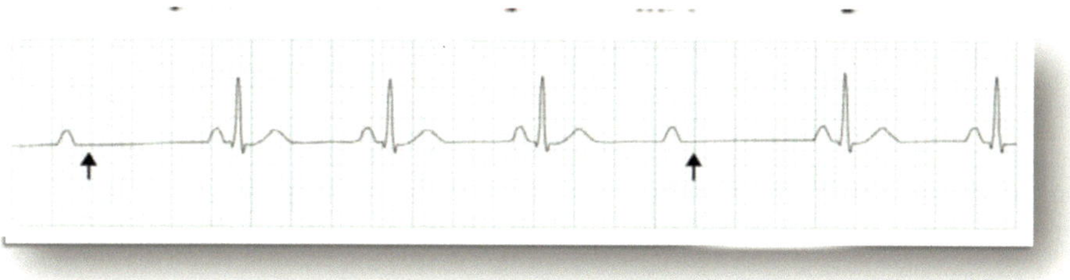

Clinical Significance

- More likely than Mobitz I to be associated with *haemodynamic compromise, severe bradycardia* and *progression to 3rd degree heart block*
- *Haemodynamic instability* may be sudden and unexpected or sudden cardiac death
- The risk of *asystole is around 35% per year*
- Cardiac monitoring required: *ultimately insertion of a permanent pacemaker*

Third Degree

Definition

- Complete absence of AV conduction: no supraventricular impulses are conducted to the ventricles
- Perfusing rhythm is maintained by a junctional or ventricular escape rhythm. Alternatively, the patient may suffer ventricular standstill leading to syncope (if self-terminating) or sudden cardiac death (if prolonged)

- Typically the patient will have severe bradycardia with independent atrial and ventricular rates, i.e. AV dissociation

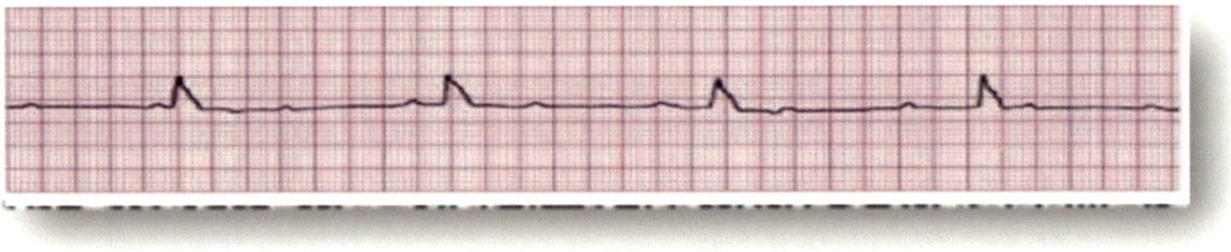

Clinical Significance

- *High risk of ventricular standstill* and *sudden cardiac death*
- Require urgent admission for cardiac monitoring, backup temporary pacing and usually *insertion of a permanent pacemaker*

Hypothermia

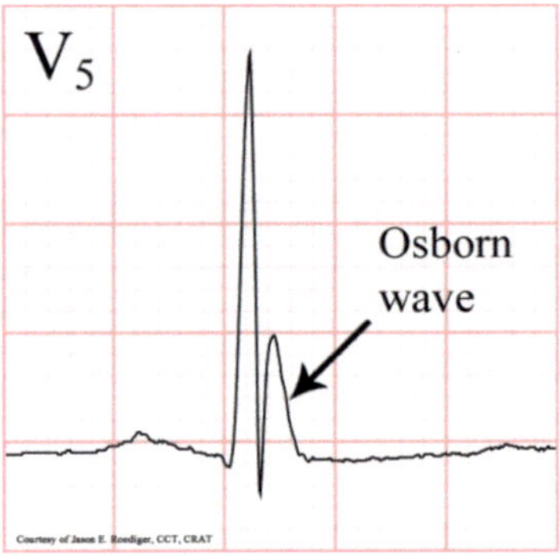

"J- waves or Osborne Waves"

Neurogenic shock

Neurogenic shock occurs after an *injury to the spinal cord*

Mechanism

- Sympathetic (autonomic pathways) outflow is disrupted resulting in unopposed vagal tone (decreased systemic vascular resistance)
- May lead to hypothermia and loss of temperature regulation

Clinical Presentation

- *Hypotension and bradycardia*. Patients are usually hypotensive with warm, dry skin
- The higher the level of injury, the more likely it is for the patient to exhibit severe symptoms
- Patients are often hypoxic and could have organ failure due to decreased blood profusion

Treatment

- Isotonic Crystalloid IV fluids should be given
- *Vasopressin agents* such as ADH and *Vasopressors* (Norepinephrine) should be used to retain fluid volume
- *Dopamine* or *Dobutamine* is used when there has been an inadequate response to volume resuscitation as they are inotropes.
- (*Phenylephrine*) is first line for those who don't respond to Dopamine
- Severe bradycardia may need to be treated with *Atropine*

Heat stroke

Definition

- Life-threatening form of heat illness than typically occurs in patients with a core temp of greater than 41C (**106F**)
- High core temperatures cause a loss of thermoregulation, tissue damage, and multisystem failure
- *Neurologic dysfunction* is the *hallmark of heat stroke* and is frequently associated with *cerebral edema*

Clinical Presentation

- Patients present very dehydrated (with very dry skin), and may exhibit confusion, disorientation, ataxia, psychosis, seizures, unconsciousness, and hemodynamic instability

Treatment

- Intensive care monitoring, blood chemistry analysis, rehydration, and rapid body cooling. Preferred method for rapid cooling is *ice water immersion*.
- *Evaporative cooling* using cold-water mists and fans may be effective

- *IV fluids* should be initiated at a rate that ensures adequate urine output, beginning with 250 mL/h NS

Heat exhaustion

Definition

- This can be life-threatening and results from dehydration and body salt depletion

Clinical Presentation

- The illness typically manifests itself as sweating, weakness, fatigue, headache, nausea, dizziness, muscle cramps and tachycardia (*sign of dehydration*). Core body temperature may be only slightly elevated and is usually less than 40C (**104F**)

Treatment

- Milder cases may respond well to *oral salt solutions*. More severe cases require hospitalization, blood chemistry and analysis, and IV rehydration.

  If left untreated can *progress to heat stroke*

Heat Syncope

Definition

- Temporary loss of consciousness caused by *brain hypoperfusion* and results from the relative *hypotension* created by peripheral vasodilation and vascular leak

Risk Factors

- Dehydration is a disposing factor

Treatment

- Condition resolves with rehydration and sitting in supine position with legs raised

Heat Rash (Prickly Heat)

Definition

- Results from *blocking of sweat gland pore* and is frequently associated with *staph infection*

Clinical Presentation

- Typically *pruritic vesicles on an erythematous base* on clothed areas of the skin and may take weeks to completely resolve

Treatment

- Topical chlorhexidine antibacterial cream, 1% salicylic acid for small areas, and oral antibiotics for more severe manifestations

Orbital Blowout Fracture

Definition

- Fracture of the orbital floor or medial wall, typically results from traumatic impact of a blunt object larger than the orbital aperture, or eye socket

Cause

- Occurs when an object of small diameter strikes the globe without causing an orbital ridge fracture
- Adipose tissue, the inferior rectus, or the inferior oblique can then *herniate* and *become entrapped* within the maxillary or ethmoid sinus
- A significant consequence is *entrapment of the inferior rectus muscle and/or orbital fat ("Teardrop sign")*
- On (*Water's view radiograph)* a fat mass can be observed hanging from the floor into the maxillary antrum "*teardrop sign*"
- This herniated mass consists of orbital contents

Clinical Presentation

- Ischemia and subsequent loss of muscle function may occur as the result of edema and hemorrhage of muscle and *extra-ocular fat* that have prolapsed through the fracture into the maxillary sinus

- If patient is asked to raise both eyes towards the ceiling and the *inferior rectus muscle is entrapped*, the affected eye will stay facing forward and will not be able to look up
- **Enophthalmos** (posterior displacement of the eyeball within the orbit) can occur

Physical Exam

- Infraorbital anesthesia often occurs with fracture of the orbital floor
- Orbital dystopia (the eye on the affected side is lower in the horizontal plane than the other) may occur because entrapped muscle and orbital fat pull the eye downward. *Diplopia* with upward gaze; decreased eye movements
- *Injury to the infra-orbital nerve* may occur, resulting in decreased sensation along the cheek, upper lip, or upper gingiva

Imaging

- *Coronal CT*: to localize the fracture

Treatment

- Prophylactic oral antibiotics to cover sinus pathogens are generally recommended for patients with orbital fractures into a sinus: Azithromycin or Augmentin
- Give appropriate *tetanus prophylaxis* and avoid valsalva.
- Sleep with HOB elevated; cold packs may be applied for first 48 hours to reduce swelling

Consult with *Ophthamology*

CK-MB

- This is a cardiac marker for acute MI
- *B subunit is specific for myocardial damage*
- Performed at admission, *8, 16 and 24* hours
- This marker has been replaced by troponin now, but useful for detecting re-infarction. CK-MB also found in skeletal muscle
- Males < 6.7 and Females <3.8= normal

Wrist drop

Definition

- A condition where a person *cannot extend their wrist* and it hangs flaccidly

"Radial nerve palsy"

Treatment

- Splint the wrist to treat initially
- Physiotherapy or occupational therapy may be indicated

Central Retinal Artery Occlusion

Definition

- Flow of blood through the central retinal artery is blocked (occluded). There are several different causes of this occlusion; the most common is *carotid artery atherosclerosis*

Clinical Presentation

- MC *Painless unilateral vision loss*
- Fundoscopic exam will show a red lesion, called a "*cherry red spot*," with surrounding *pale retina* (the pale color is caused by ischemia of the retina)

Treatment

- *Hyperbaric oxygen therapy*, ocular massage, anterior chamber paracentesis, and inhalation therapy of a mixture of 5% carbon dioxide and 95% oxygen

Appendicitis Tests

Psoas Sign

- Passively extend thigh while patient is lying on their side with knees extended
- If pain results, psoas sign is positive OR if pain in abdomen with flexion of right knee against resistance

Obturator Sign

- Pain with internal rotation of thigh with hip flexed at 90 degrees

Rovsing Sign

- Palpation of the left lower quadrant of a person's abdomen increases the pain felt in the right lower quadrant, the patient is said to have a positive Rovsing's sign and may have appendicitis

Cholecystitis

- Murphy's sign
- US is test of choice- can also be indicative of pancreatitis

McBurney Point

- (1/3 of distance from iliac crest to umbilicus)

Treatment: Appendectomy is definitive

> **Parkland formula**
>
> (fluid replacement for burns in first 24 hours)= (4 x kg) x % BSA
>
> First half is delivered in 8 hours, remaining in last 16 hours.

Mallet Finger

Definition

- Difficulty extending *DIP joint*: (baseball finger, dropped finger, dolphin finger) or extensor tendon injury caused by blunt force

Burns

Rule of 9's

- 9% for each arm
- 18% for each each leg
- 18% front of the torso
- 18% back of the torso
- 9% head
- 1% perineum

Animal and Human Bites

Treatment

- Irrigate wound with NS or tap water (shown to be just as effective)

Cat bites: P. multocida

Medications

- Amoxicillin/Clavulanate (Augmentin) 875 mg PO BID x 5-10days + tetanus and consider rabies prophylaxis
- For higher-risk infections, a first dose of antibiotic may be given intravenously (ampicillin-sulbactam, ticarcillin-clavulanate, piperacillin-tazobactam, or a carbapenem)
- For *Monkey bites* give prophylactic acyclovir for 14 days

Bacteria

- (MC) Pasteurella multocida
- Common organisms include capnocytophagia canimorsus, pasteurella, staphylococcus, streptococcus

Nephrolithiasis

Presentation

- Acute onset of *severe flank pain radiating to the groin*, gross or *microscopic hematuria*, *nausea*, and *vomiting* not associated with an acute abdomen are symptoms that most likely indicate renal colic caused by an acute ureteral or renal pelvic obstruction from a calculus

Imaging

- *Non-contrast CT scan* is gold standard
- **Abdominal plain film**: monitor passage (large stones only), intravenous pyelography
- **IVP**: more for degree of obstruction
- **Ultrasound:** is used for young patients and pregnant women

Treatment

- **Less than 5mm:** Pass spontaneously + fluids and analgesics (NSAIDs or opioids).
- **5mm to 10mm**: May pass spontaneously, but less likely the bigger they are
- **11 to 20 mm**: Shockwave lithotripsy
- **>2 cm**: Percutaneous nephrolithotomy or open surgery

Pneumothorax

Tension: Needs to be treated with *emergent needle decompression* at the second intercostal space and *chest tube*

Clinical Presentation

- Chest pain, SOB, tachycardia, tachypnea, unilateral decreased breath sounds, displaced trachea. MC due to trauma of the chest

Imaging

- Chest x-ray to diagnose small PTX

Spontaneous

Primary: *No underlying lung disease*

- Risk factors include smoking, male, and family history of PTX

Secondary: *Underlying lung disease present*

- Risk Factors: COPD, severe asthma, TB, Sarcoidosis, connective tissue disorder like Marfan's syndrome (tall, thin, long limbs), lung cancer
- (*Tall skinny males=MC*)

Pancreatitis

Definition

- Inflammation of the pancreas. (*MC) due to ETOH or Cholelithiasis.*
- Can involve the release of pancreatic enzymes in which are abnormally activated in the pancreas and can *auto-digest the functional pancreatic cells*

Clinical Presentation

- *Abdominal pain*, which is characteristically dull, boring, and steady
- Pain is *sudden in onset* and gradually intensifies in severity until reaching a constant ache
- MC located in the upper abdomen, usually in the *Epigastric region*, but it may be perceived more on the left or right side, depending on which portion of the pancreas is involved
- The pain radiates directly through the *abdomen to the back* in approximately one half of cases

Physical exam findings

- Tender epigastrium, may be distended, hypoactive bowel sounds
- Could have *scleral icterus* due to Choledocholithiasis
- May have fever, tachypnea, hypoxemia, and hypotension in severe cases

Key signs

Cullen's sign: Ecchymosis in paraumbilical region
Grey-Turner's sign: Ecchymosis along the flank

Labs

Amylase: Increases in 6-12 hours

- Greater than 3 x normal indicates pancreatitis

Lipase: (**Most Specific**) increases in 4-8 hours

- Elevations last longer than amylase elevations
- CRP, TNF are also elevated in pancreatitis

May find leukocytosis, elevated hematocrit, BUN, hypocalcaemia, hyperglycemia, and hypoglycemia

Imaging

Contrast Abdominal CT

- Focal or diffuse enlargement of pancreas with heterogeneous enhancement of contrast. Necrosis is seen as lack of enhancement of contrast

Ultrasound

- Diffuse enlargement and hypoechoic

Abdominal X-rays

- Potential localized ileus or colon cutoff sign in more severe cases (no air distal to splenic flexure)
- Ground glass appearance may be from peripancreatic fluid collection

Treatment

- First line Tx involves *Fluid resuscitation* (NS or LR), *pain control* (IV opioids like Fentanyl) and *nutritional support* if severe
- Monitor electrolytes (hypocalcaemia, hyperglycemia, hypoglycemia)

Abx ONLY if septic, UTI or pneumonia develop

GI Bleeding

Upper

Hematemesis and/or melena in vomit (MC)

- **Esophageal varices**: d/t portal hypertension from liver cirrhosis, jaundice, weakness, fatigue, anorexia, abdominal distention
- **Esophageal ulcer**: Odynophagia, GERD, dysphagia
- **Mallory-Weiss tear:** Emesis, retching, coughing prior to emesis
- **Peptic Ulcer disease:** H. pylori history, NSAID use, smoking, epigastric or RUQ pain
    - *Duodenal- better with food*
    - *Gastric- worse with food*
- **Malignancy:** Smoking, alcohol abuse, H. pylori infection, dysphagia, early satiety, involuntary weight loss, cachexia

Lower

Hematochezia (Blood in stool)

- **Diverticulosis:** MC, Older age, *painless,* large volume blood loss-diagnose via colonoscopy
- **Inflammatory bowel disease:** Diarrhea, crampy abdominal pain, fever, fatigue
- **Crohns**: Affects *anywhere* from *mouth to anus*. Can also affect skin, eyes, joints and liver. Symptoms worse after eating. *Ulcers and fistulas form*.

- **Ulcerative Colitis:** *Colon only*. Only affects *superficial layers of bowel*. Urgent bowel.
- **Infectious diarrhea:** Bloody diarrhea, abdominal pain, fever, dehydration, e. coli, c diff, shigella, campylobacter, salmonella
- **Malignancy:** Polyps, older age, weight loss, etc.
- **Hemorrhoids, anal fissures, rectal ulcers**: Minor bleeding, itching, internal are painless, blood drips into toilet or coats stool

FAST Exam

Definition

- Focused Assessment with sonography for trauma. Performed to look for *abnormal fluid (blood) in four areas*

    - **Morison pouch** (hepatorenal)
    - **Splenorenal recess**
    - **Pouch of Douglas** (pelvis-rectouterine pouch)
    - **Pericardium** (Subxiphoid). Can also look for hemothorax bilaterally.

Meningitis

Definition

- An acute inflammation of the protective membranes covering the brain and spinal cord, known as the meninges

Clinical Presentation

- *Nuchal rigidity* is a sign of meningeal irritation
- *Kernig's sign*: Pain in the neck or back when a pt with meningitis attempts to extend the leg at the knee while the thigh is held in 90 degrees of flexion
- *Brudzinski's sign*: Spontaneous flexion of the hips during attempted passive flexion of the neck
- *Petechia or Pupura* MC with N. Meningitidis

All patients with focal neurologic deficit, papilledema, or alteration in mental status should undergo *CT of the head* to *rule out mass lesion before LP*.

- If there is to be a delay in performing an LP, empiric antibiotics must be started immediately, ideally within 30 minutes of the patient's arrival in the ED.

CSF Fluid characteristics

- Bacterial Meningitis: Opening pressure >300 mmHg, >1000 WBCs, <40 mg/dL glucose, >200 mg/dL protein, + gram stain and culture.
- Viral Meningitis: Opening pressure <200 mmHg, <1000 WBCs, >40 mg/dL glucose, <200 mg/dL protein, - gram stain and culture.

Treatment

- **Neonates:** Ampicillin and Ceftriaxone
- **1-3 months:** Ampicillin, Ceftriaxone, and Dexamethasone
- **3 months-50 years**: Ceftriaxone, Vancomycin, and Dexamethasone
- **>50 years or alcohol**: Ampicillin, Ceftriaxone, Dexamethasone

Glasgow Coma Scale

($E_4V_5M_6$)

Eye opening: Max (4)

- Spontaneous→4 points
- To verbal commands→3 points
- To painful stimuli→2 points
- To response→1 point

Verbal response: Max (5)

- Oriented and alert→5 points
- Disoriented conversation→4 points
- Speaking but non-sensical→3 points
- Incomprehensible sounds→2 points
- No response→1 point

Motor response: Max (6)

- Follows commands→6 points
- Localizes pain→5 points
- Moves or withdraws to pain→4 points
- Decorticate flexion (to core)→3 points
- Decerebrate extension (indicates higher up lesion)→2 points
- No response→1 point

Total out of 15----- 7 or less needs to be intubated

Antidotes for Intoxications

Sedative-hypnotic

- Decreased level of consciousness, bradypnea, respiratory depression, hypotension, miosis
- Caused by opiates, ethanol, benzos, barbiturates

Anticholinergic

- Tachycardia, pyrexia, dry mouth, mydriasis, flushed skin. Usually caused by antihistamines (OTC diphenhydramine-benadryl)

Cholinergic

- Salivation, lacrimation, urination, diarrhea, GI distress and emesis. Usually caused by agricultural exposure to organophosphate-based pesticides

Sympathomimetic

- HTN, tachycardia, mydriasis, arrhythmias. Caused by amphetamines, meth, cocaine, ectasy.

Overdose on acetaminophen

- Activated charcoal. **NAC (N-acetyl cysteine)** is antidote.

Overdose on salicylates

- **Activated charcoal**. Urinary alkalization with sodium bicarbonate promotes renal elimination of salicylates.

Overdose on anticholinergic

- **Physiostigmine** (cholinesterase inhibitor)

Digoxin toxicity

- Increases myocardial contractility and slow electrical conduction at the AV node. Present w bradycardia, hypotension.

Overdose on opiates

- **Narcan** (naloxone)

PCN Adverse Reactions

- Steven Johnson Syndrome
- Erythema multiform→target lesions

Anaphylaxis

Definition

- Anaphylaxis is a Type I hypersensitivity reactions that occurs in previously sensitized individuals
- **Initial exposure** to an allergen, IgE antibodies are formed and bind to mast cells or basophils
- **On subsequent re-exposure**, the antigen combines with the IgE antibodies bound to mast cells or basophils, causing release of chemical mediators

Clinical Manifestations

- Caused by the release of these chemical mediators
  - Histamine, leukotrienes, prostaglandins, and platelet-activating factor
  - These mediators produce vasodilation, increased vascular permeability, and smooth muscle spasm, resulting in

hypotension, urticarial, bronchospasm, and angioedema of the skin, upper airway, and GI tract

Requires sensitization first→after exposure the B cells switch from IgG and IgM production to IgE.

Clinical Presentation

- The skin or mucous membranes are involved in 80-90% of cases
- **Local rxn**: Swelling, pain, itching
- **Systemic rxn**: Whole body itching (ears, mouth, tongue, throat, scalp), urticaria, angioedema of lips, tongue, face, wheezing or dyspnea (swelling causes obstruction and difficulty breathing)

Treatment

Epinephrine (IM) "First line recommended"

- H_1 blockers
- Beta agonists
- Vasopressors
- Corticosteroids
- Positive inotropic agents

Suture Sizes and Durations

- Nylon, silk, polyester, polybutester, polypropylene (prolene): *Non-absorbable*
- Vicryl: *Absorbable*

More zeros: Smaller size suture

- 3-0 is bigger than 7-0

Face: 6.0 or 7.0 absorbable suture. *4-5 days to remove from face/ear*
Back, Palms and Soles: 3-0

Salter Harris Fractures

- I→**Separation** at the physis: Fracture through the growth plate
- II→**Above**: Through physis and metaphysis
- III→**Lower**: Through physis and epiphysis
- IV→**Through**: Everything (metaphysis, physis, epiphysis)
- V→**ER**: Compression fracture

Fractures of the Upper Arm

Radial Nerve→runs in bicipital groove: Often compromised
Often get wrist drop

Skull fractures

Battle sign

- Ecchymosis of mastoid process of temporal bone

Le Fort fracture

- A classic *trans facial fracture* of the mid-face, involving the maxillary bone and surrounding structures in either a horizontal, pyramidal or transverse direction
- The hallmark of Lefort fractures is *traumatic pterygomaxillary separation*, which signifies fractures between the ptergoid horseshoe shaped bony protuberances, which extend from the inferior margin of the maxilla and the maxillary sinuses

Localizing MI on an EKG

II, III, AVF = inferior MI "**ST Elevation**"

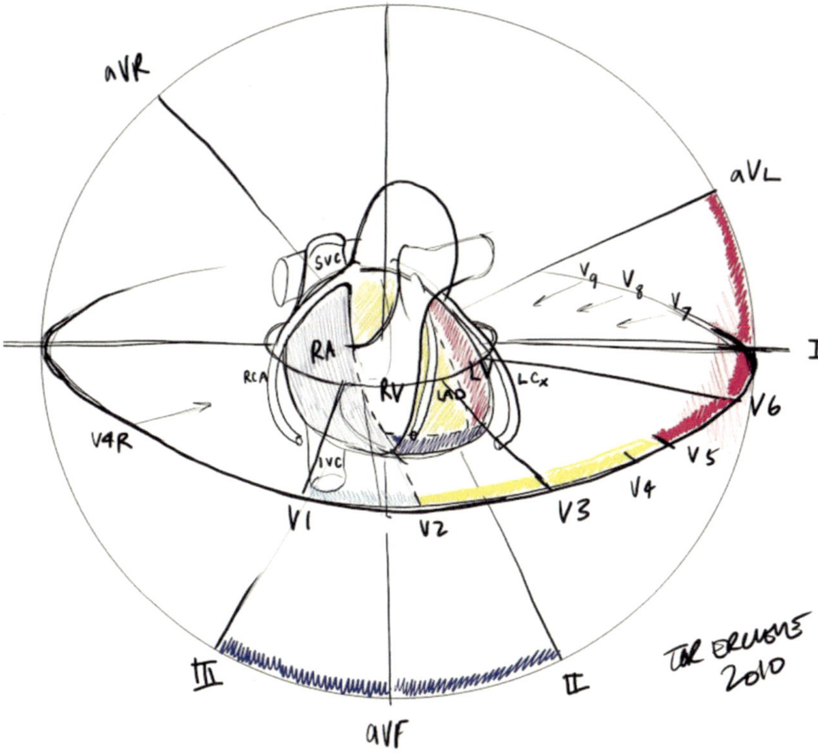

Figure 6: Image copyrighted to Tor Ecleve 2010

Abdominal Aortic Aneurism and Aortic Dissection

AAA

- True aneurysm involves all three layers (*intima, media, adventitia*)
- Patients are usually asymptomatic but may present with dull constant abdominal, low back, or flank pain

Physical Exam

- *Pulsatile mass in abdomen*. (Look with U/S)

Aortic Dissection

Physical Exam

- *Muffled heart sounds* consistent with cardiac tamponade

Imaging

- CT with contrast
- Longitudinal splitting of the arterial wall from a defect in the intimal layer

Clinical Presentation

- Severe "*tearing of abdominal pain that radiates to the back*"

Pericarditis

Definition

- Inflammation of the fibrous pericardial sac that surrounds the heart
- A pericardial effusion may be present
- The visceral layer that surrounds the epicardium and a parietal layer that surrounds the heart normally contain 15-50 mL of fluid

Severity depends on how much and rate of leak into the pericardium

Physical Exam

- " *Pericardial friction rub*", best heard with pt. leaning forward.
- Look for signs of cardiac tamponade (*Muffled heart sounds, JVD, Hypotension=**Beck's Triad***)

Pulsus Paradoxus: (fall in systolic BP >10 mmHg *with inspiration*)

Labs

- Increased urea (BUN) or increased blood creatinine in cases of uremic pericarditis

Imaging

- Echo can help diagnose

Treatment

- The treatment in viral or idiopathic pericarditis is with aspirin or *non-steroidal anti-inflammatory drugs (NSAIDs such as ibuprofen)*
- *Colchicine* may be added to the above as it decreases the risk of further episodes of pericarditis

Endocarditis

Definition

- Inflammation of the endocardium and heart valves

Complications

- **Rheumatic heart dx**: Mitral valve (vegetation's)
- **IV drug user**: Tricuspid valve or pulmonic valve
- Prosthetic heart valve

Clinical Presentation

- Fever, altered mental status and frank sepsis are common
- Fundoscopic Exam→*Roth spots*: small white spots on retina surrounded by hemorrhage
- **Osler nodes**→ *Painful lesions* that form on fat pads of fingers or toes and represent immune complex deposition
- **Janeway lesions**→*Painless lesions*, reddish, macular lesions on palms or soles of feet
- *Splinter hemorrhages* under fingernails or toenails

Treatment

- Nafcillin and gentamicin are appropriate first line treatment
- Further therapy should be guided by *culture results* and treatment should be continued for at *least 4 weeks*

Pneumonia, Pneumothorax

Pneumothorax

- Tachypnea, tachycardia, decreased breath sounds on side of the pneumothorax and hyper resonance to percussion on that side indicate ***spontaneous pneumothorax***.

- Hypotension, tracheal deviation, and elevated JVD indicate ***tension pneumo***.
- Trachea deviates to side opposite of pneumothorax

Pneumonia

- *Strep* (MC community-acquired), Staph, Haemophilus, Pseudomonas. Dullness to percussion, tactile fremitus, egophony, rales

Treatment: Levofloxacin or azithromycin

Preeclampsia/Eclampsia

Preeclampsia

- *HTN* in pregnancy associated with *proteinuria (>300 mg/day)* and *nondependent edema* (hands, face)
- Usually occurs during 3rd trimester; patients presents with sudden weight gain and notice swelling in their hands and face
- Other symptoms include HA, Epigastric pain, visual disturbances, and oliguria
- *BP >140/90* measured twice at least 6 hours apart

Eclampsia: Seizures in a pt. with preeclampsia.

HELLP Syndrome: *Hemolysis Elevated Liver Enzymes, Low Platelets.*

Treatment

Mild preeclampsia

- Deliver if term or evidence of fetal lung maturity
- Admit patient, control BP with *IV hydralazine*, *magnesium sulfate* for seizure prophylaxis

Severe preeclampsia

- Expedite delivery regardless of lung maturity if beyond 32 weeks or evidence of renal failure. Control BP with IV hydralazine
- Give *magnesium sulfate for seizure control*
- *Definitive tx is delivery of the fetus*
- All patients with preeclampsia/ eclampsia require admission

UTI and STD

UTI

Bacteria

- *(MC) E. Coli*. *Staph Sapropyticus* is MC in sexually active female teens
- Pregnant, immune-compromised, elderly may present with asymptomatic bacteremia

Labs

- Urine dip: look for leukocyte esterase (pyuria) and nitrites (bacteremia)
- UA: >10 WBC and presence of any bacteria

Treatment

- Bactrim, Cipro, Pyridium for relief (bladder anesthetic) for 3 days
  **If pyelonephritis, do same Cipro but 14 days*

Gonorrhea

- MC in *middle aged men*
- Dysuria, purulent discharge, "strawberry cervix"
- Ceftriaxone 125 mg IM x1 dose

Chlamydia

- MC in *young males*
- Clear discharge, friable erythematous cervix
- Azithromycin 1g PO X1

Syphilis

- Painless chancre is primary Syphilis
- Secondary Syphilis can present 3-6 days after primary chancre resolves
- **Clinical Presentation**: Sore throat, fever, headache. A dull, red papular rash develops on palms, soles, and trunk
- **Treatment**: penicillin G (3 does/ 1week apart)

Trichamonas

- It is a common *cause of vaginitis*
- It is a sexually transmitted infection, and is caused by the single-celled protozoan parasite Trichomonas vaginalis producing mechanical stress on host cells and then ingesting cell fragments after cell death
- **Treatment**: Metronidazole 2g

Recombinant TPA Therapy

- Due to lack of pain fibers within the brain parenchyma, ischemic strokes typically do not cause a headache
- This is in contrast with a hemorrhagic stroke, which do cause headaches due to the irritating effects of blood on the dura
    - In an *ischemic stroke*, BP is frequently elevated as a result of brain's auto regulation of cerebral vasculature. *HTN after ischemic stroke should not be treated unless severe (>220/>120)*
    - HTN in stroke usually tx with nitroprusside.
    - IV thrombolytics (tPA) should be considered in patients presenting with ischemic strokes of ***< 3 hours*** duration and no evidence of hemorrhage on CT scan

Primary Treatment of DKA (fruity breath)

- Fluids 4-6x Maintenance (Volume depletion), insulin, and bicarb to push potassium intracellular. Also if K+ is normal or decreased give K+

SIRS Criteria

Meet 2 or more of the following

Temp	>38 or 104 or <36
Heart Rate	>90
RR	>20 or $PaCO_2$<32 mm Hg
WBC	>12,000 or <4000 or >10% bands

Sepsis Criteria: (Cunha, B., MD. 2016)

- Must meet SIRS criteria + suspected source or present source of infection

Severe Sepsis

- Organ dysfunction, Hypotension or Hypo profusion
- Lactic Acidosis
- SBP <90 or SBP drop >40mm Hg from normal

Severe Septic Shock

- Severe Sepsis with hypotension, despite adequate fluid resuscitation

Multiple Organ Dysfunction Syndromes

- Evidence of >2 organs failing

Chapter Seven

Gynecology

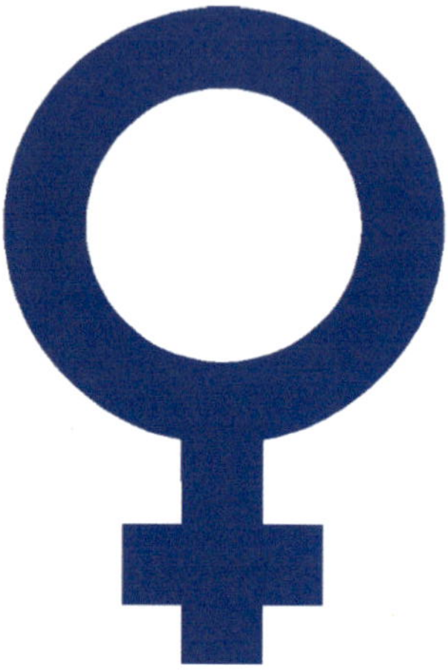

Sexually Transmitted Infections/ GU issues

Chlamydia

- MC bacterial STD in US

Etiology

- Chlamydia trachomatis: causes ocular, respiratory, and reproductive tract infections

Method of transmission

- Sexual contact
- Vertical transmission: from mother to newborn

Clinical manifestation

- Asymptomatic common
- Cervicitis, urethriti, and PID

Diagnosis

- Gold Standard: Tissue culture of endocervical canal
- Rotate swab deep in endocervical canal for 15-20 seconds
- PCR or DNA probe

Treatment:

- Doxycycline 100mg BID for 7 days or
- Azithromycin 1g PO in a single dose

Trichomoniasis

- Unicellular flagellated protozoon that inhabits vagina and lower urinary tract
- MC nonviral, nonchlamydial STD of women

Method of transmission

- Sexual contact

Clinical Manifestation

- *Asymptomatic* is common
- Profuse vaginal discharge
- Frothy white, gray, yellow, or GRAY-GREEN
- Unpleasant odor
- Puritis
- Dysuria and urinary frequency
- Vulvar and labial swelling
- Cervical petechiae: "Strawberry Cervix"

Symptoms

- Worse immediately after menses because of the transient increase in vaginal pH
- Protozoon seen on saline wet prep
- Positive whiff test—KOH--- amine odor release from cells
- Vaginal pH= >5.0

Treatment

- Metronidazole: 2g PO one dose or 500mg BID 7 days both partners or
- Requires hepatic metabolism
- Side effects: N/V, metallic taste, inhibits alcohol metabolism
- Tinidazole 2g PO one dose

Genital Herpes

- Most prevalent genital ulcer: 80% unaware

Primary Infections

- Flulike symptoms: malaise, myalgias, nausea, diarrhea, and fever
- Vulvar burning and puritis
- Multiple vesicles that last for 24-36 hrs. Before turning into painful genital ulcers
- Recurrent episodes can occur frequently
- Women should have a vaginal exam around the time of delivery. Women with lesions at this time must delivery baby via cesarean

Diagnosis

- Examination of vesicles and ulcers
- Sexual history
- Viral cultures are gold standard for diagnosis
- Viral serology: IgG for primary lesion, IgM for recurrence

Treatment

- No cure
- Primary infection: acyclovir 200 mg for 5 times per day for 7 to 10 days or
- Famiciclovir, valcyvlovir
- Recurrent infection: prophylactic or suppression therapy of 400mg orally twice a day

HPV

- Genital warts usually caused by HPV 6 and 11
- HPV 16, 18 cause 70% of cervical cancers

Method of transmission

- Sexual contact
- Transmission can occur even if lesion free
- Pregnancy: Condylomata increase in number and size
- Transmission from mom to infant is rare
- No podophyllin or Imiquimod or podofilox

Clinical manifestations

- Majority is latent with no visible lesions
- Condylomata: verrucous fleshy papules that may coalesce into plaques
- Lesions typically appear within weeks to months after exposure
- May include pruritis, burning, bleeding, dyspareunia

Diagnosis

- Clinical exam
- Application of acetic acid causes wart to turn white

Treatment

- Local excision, cryotherapy, topical trichloroacetic acid (TCA), topical phodophyllin, 5-fluorouracil
- Need to be repeated weekly till all lesions are gone
- TCA is approved for pregnancy
- Larger condylomas: CO2 laser may be used to vaporize lesion

Syphilis

- The spirochete Treponema pallidum cause the chronic systemic infection

Method of transmission

- Sexual contact
- Mother to baby
- Spirochete enters the body through a small abrasion in the skin or mucosal surface and replicates locally

Clinical manifestations

Moderately contagious—MC first 2 years

- Infectious during the primary, secondary, and first year of latent phase
- Latent phase—2-20yrs

Three phases

- **Primary syphilis**
  - Painless, red, round, firm ulcer—chancre
  - Heals spontaneously in 2-6 wks
  - 50% progress to secondary phase, 50% latent

- **Secondary syphilis**
  - Hematogenous spread of spirocehetes—bacteremia
  - Maculopapular rash classically found on palms and soles
  - Condyloma lantum
  - (Large raised flattened grayish, white areas) develops 6wks to 6 mo. after primary chancre)

- Painless lymphadenopathy

- **Tertiary syphilis**
  - Characterized by granulomas (gummas) of skin and bones
  - Cardiovascular syphilis with aortitis
  - Neurosyphilis with meningovascular disease, paresis, and tabes dorsalis (neuropathy)

Diagnosis

Two types of non-treponemal serologic test (nonspecific) for syphilis:

- **VDRL:** Venereal disease research labs
- **RPR:** Rapid plasma regain
  - These tests remain positive for 6 to 12 months after tx of primary syphilis
  - Antitreponemal antibody: specific

- **FTA-ABA:** fluorescent treponemal antibody absorption
- **TPPA:** treponema pallidum particle agglutination assay

Treatment

Penicillin G IV or tetracycline/doxycline if allergic

- Jarish-herxheimer rxn
- Worse with within 24 hrs of PCN
  - Fever, chills, HA, myalgia, malaise, pharyngitis, rash
  - Might induce preterm labor
  - *Good sign* susceptible to treatment
- Treatment after first phase: need negative nonspecific serology with in first year
- Treatment after second phase: need negative serology with 2 years

If not negative, treatment failure, reinfection, concurrent infection with HIV

Gonorrhea

Neisseria gonorrhea (gram negative diplococcic bacteria) is responsible

Method of transmission

- Sexual contact

Clinical manifestations

- Majority are asymptomatic
- Mucopurulent cervicitis, swollen/red/friable cervix, acute urethritis
- PID
- Bartholin abscess

Diagnosis

- Culture via Thayer-martin agar

Treatment

- Ceftriaxone 125mg IM once, or Cefixime 400 mg orally 1x

Candidiasis

- Caused by Candida Albicans
- Chronic infections: >4 episodes a year (think HIV, DM)
- NOT an STD

Clinical Manifestations

- Pruritis, Vulvar burning, Dysuria burning, Dysparunia, Vaginal discharge, Erythema
- Edema, Excoriations, White/gray/viscous/granular vaginal discharge

Diagnosis

- No odor (-whiff)
- pH< 4.5
- **Wet prep:** Candida Albicans forms spores and hyphae (*spaghetti and meat balls*)

Treatment

Uncomplicated: Azoles

- Vaginal suppository/vulvar cream
- Oral azoles contraindicated in pregnancy, can give topial
- Note: azoles are oil based and weaken latex condoms and diaphragms

Chronic

- Azoles for long term
- 5 day treatment check LFT's
- Vulvar hygiene

Chancroid

Caused by Haemophilus Ducreyi

- STD more common in the tropics and Southeast Asia
- Cofactor for HIV transmission
- Coinfection with syphilis and HSV

Clinical manifestation

- Painful, demarcated, non-indurated ulcer
- Inguinal lymphadenopathy

Diagnosis

- H. ducreyi is difficult to culture
- Dx usually made clinically

Treatment

- Ceftriaxone 250 mg IM once or
- Azithromycin 1g PO once or
- Ciprofloxacin 500 mg PO twice a day for 3 days or
- Erythromycin 500 mg 4 times a day for 7 days
- *Treat partners*

Bacterial Vaginosis:

Occurs with a shift in predominate bacterial species in vagina.

- One common causative organism is Gardnerella Vaginalis
- Leading cause of vaginitis
- Not an STD

Clinical Manifestations

- Grey/white, malodorous, creamy, non-inflammatory vaginal discharge
- Little to no vulvar irritation or pruritus

Diagnosis

- **Saline wet prep and** gram stain reveal: Clue cells
- (+) whiff test
- pH >4.5

Treatment

- Metronidazole 500 mg PO BID for 7 days or
- Single dose of 2 g PO metronidazole
- Metronidazole vaginal gel
- In pregnancy treatment of choice is metronidazole 250 mg PO TID for 7 days (second and third trimester)
- Clindamycin is *not recommended*

Leiomyoma

- Also called fibroids or uterine myomas
- Benign proliferations of smooth muscle cell of the myometrium
- Most common pelvic tumor in women
- Typically occur in women of child bearing age and then regress

Pathogenesis

- Estrogen effect is questionable
- A Myomatous uterus has an increased number of arteries and veins

Fibroid location

- Intramural: Within uterine wall

Most common type

Sub-mucosal

- Derive from myometrial cells just below endometrium
  - Often protrude into uterine cavity

Sub-serosal

- Just under serosal surface of uterus and has a broad orpedunculated base
- May (extend between folds of the broad ligament)

Cervical fibroids:

- In cervix rather than uterus
- Not in prepubertal girls
- OCP, parity, smoking, and consumption of green vegetables are *protective* against fibroids

Risk factors

- Early menarche, Early exposure to OCP, Significant consumption of beef, ham or other red meats, HTN, Family predisposition, Uterine infection and being African American.

Clinical Manifestations

- Increased uterine bleeding (NOT intermenstrual)
- Pelvic pressure and pain
- Reproductive dysfunction
- Symptoms related to number, size, and location
- Relief of symptoms at the time of menopause
- Bimanual exam reveals non-tender irregularly enlarged uterus (lumpy and bumpy)

Diagnosis

- Transvaginal US:

- Saline infusion sonography: Tells extent of protrusion into endometrial cavity
    - Identifies lesions not identified on US
- Hysterosalpingography (HSG): Defines contour of the endometrial cavity
- MRI: visualizing size and location of all uterine myomas

Treatment

Most cases do not require treatment

Patients with actively growing fibroids should be followed every 6 months

Progesterone only contraceptives: causes endometrial atrophy

- Gonadotropin-releasing hormone (GnRH) agonists: *most effective*
- Ultimately puts patients in postmenopausal state
- Anti-progestin mifepristone (RU-486): reduces uterine volume
- Levonorgestrel: reduces uterine volume and bleeding
- Myomectomy: removal of fibroid
- Endometrial ablation: used in women who have completed childbearing
- Uterine artery embolization: effective option for women who wish to preserve their uterus and not interested in future fertility
- Hysterectomy: main advantage is that it eliminates current symptoms and chance for recurrence

Lichen sclerosis

Definition

This is a benign, chronic, inflammatory process and the most common vulvar dermatologic disorder

- White thickening/patches around the vulva

Evaluation

- *White, atrophic papules* may coalesce into porcelain-white plaques and lead to labia minora regression, clitoral concealment, urethral obstruction, and introital stenosis

Lab Testing

- A consistent relationship between lichen sclerosus and autoimmune disorders
- Vulvar Biopsy to exclude pre-invasive and invasive lesions

Management

First line: Topical corticosteroid

- Clobetasol propionate 0.05%, twice daily for 1 month and then daily for 3 months, has been shown to be most effective for treatment of lichen sclerosus, with approximately 75% success.
- A subsequent taper to lower-potency topical steroids is necessary for maintenance of therapy.

Other options

- Oral antihistamine agent can be given at bedtime for itching
- Alternative therapies: include tacrolimus cream, retinoids, cryotherapy, antimalarial agents, and photodynamic therapy.
- Surgical therapy: limited to treatment of introital narrowing, pseudocysts, and associated squamous cell carcinoma
- Vulvar hygiene
- Avoid using gels, scented bath products, moisturizing wipes, and soaps, as they may contain irritants
- Use aqueous creams to clean the vulva
- Dab the vulva gently to dry
- Avoid wearing tight fitting pants
- White cotton underwear is preferred
- Consider wearing skirts and no underwear when in the house and at night to avoid friction and aid drying

Endometriosis

Cyclic pelvic pain

"Key words"

- Barbed wire pain
- Chocolate cysts
- Mulberry raspberry cysts

- Afebrile

Triad symptoms

- Pelvic pain with Firm fixed, tender, adenexal mass

Tender nodularity

- Cul-de sac, Posterior vaginal fornix or uterosacral

Diagnosis

- Direct visualization with laparoscopy or laparotomy
  - Must see: endometrial glands, stroma, and hemosiderin-laden macs

Treatment

No role for medication in young patients trying to conceive
Laparoscopic or open surgery for women desiring future pregnancies

- Destroy all implants and remove all adhesions
- Endometriosis >3 cm – surgical resection
- Endometriosis <3 cm – laser ablation

Radical Treatment:
TAH/BSO/ LND

Polycystic Ovarian Cysts

Symptoms

- Cutaneous hyperandrogenism
- Menstrual irregularity
- Oligo or amenorrhea, or irregular bleeding
- Polycystic ovaries
- Obesity and insulin resistance
- Often have hirtusim, Acanthos nigricnas- darkening of the skin folds, elevated adrenal androgen

Cervical Cancer

HPV 16, 18 most common cause of cervical cancer

Presentation

- Abnormal vaginal bleeding, Postcoital bleeding, Pelvic pain, dyspareunia, Cervical mass, Cervical bleeding
- Locally advanced disease may present with bleeding, discharge, pain, or obstructive uropathy
- Mucoid or purulent vaginal discharge
- Bladder, renal, or bowel obstruction
- Bone pain

Risk Factors

- Age 45 to 49 years
- HPV infection, HIV
- Early onset of sexual activity (younger than 18), Multiple sexual partners, Cigarette smoking, Immunosuppression

Diagnosis

- Vaginal or speculum examination
- Colposcopy
- Biopsy
- HPV testing
- Pap smear screening followed by colposcopy may dx pre-invasive disease
- Staging is clinical, and does not incorporate lymph node evaluation or imaging results, but uses MRI to evaluate local extent of disease, and PET to screen for metastases

Treatment

- Pre-invasive disease (**carcinoma in situ**)
  - Loop electrosurgical excision or colonization
- Early stage invasive disease:
  - Surgery
- Locally advanced disease:
  - Chemo radiation therapy is significantly superior to radiation therapy alone.

Post-Menopausal Bleeding

Presentation

- Any bleeding that occurs more than 12 months after the last menstrual period, it is always abnormal
- **MCC of postmenopausal bleeding is endometrial and/or vaginal atrophy *not cancer* (CA is responsible for 10-15% of all postmenopausal bleeding**

Evaluation

Careful inspection of the external anogenital region, vulva, vagina, and cervix, a pap smear should be performed as well as a DRE and occult blood screening

Tests

- CBC, TSH, prolactin, and FSH levels, and if an ovarian mass is identified tumor markers (LDH, hCG, AFP, CEA, inhibin, and estradiol) should be considered
- **Endometrial biopsy**: Even if there is an identifiable source of post-menopausal bleeding
- **Pelvic ultrasound, sonohysterogram, and MRI**
    - An endometrial stripe (should be $\leq$ 3 mm) in postmenopausal women and uterine cavity
    - Hysteroscopy can evaluate for intrauterine abnormalities such as endometrial polyps and fibroids

D&C is both *diagnostic and therapeutic* for some lesions of the uterus and cervix

Birth Control and Oral Contraceptives

Most Effective: Hormonal IUD or Implantable Rod

The *Mirena* has a *0.1%* failure (*Most widely used reversible contraception in the world*)

- **Complications:** if pregnancy does occur with one in place the spontaneous abortion rate is 40-50%

- **Side effects:** can have pain and bleeding, expulsion, perforation, or infection; women can get insertion-related PID if they have cervical infections prior to IUD placement

Least Effective

- Spermicides alone and condoms: Failure rate is 29%
- Complications: placed in the vagina 30 minutes before intercourse, messy to use, may make users *more susceptible* to STIs and HIV by causing vaginal irritation
- Should not be used by women with HIV or at high risk of contracting it
- Side effects: Can irritate the vaginal mucosa and external genital

Contraindications

- Thrombophlebitis or thromboembolic disorders
- Cerebro-vascular or coronary artery disease
- Carcinoma of the breast or other estrogen-dependent neoplasia
- Undiagnosed abnormal genital bleeding
- Known or suspected pregnancy
- Benign or malignant liver tumor

Ovarian Cancer

Presentation

- Average age is 60 yrs. Old
- Pelvic mass, GI sx, Sx>3 months, Ascites, Abdominal distention

Risk Factors

- BRCA1 mutation, BRCA2 mutation , Increasing age , family history of ovarian cancer , Family history of breast cancer , Never used OCP , Lynch II syndrome
- Other: Nulliparity, obesity

Diagnosis

- Pelvic US: presence of solid, complex, septated, multiloculated mass; high blood flow
- CT scan: peritoneal thickening, enlarged lymph nodes, ascites, omental thickening, liver metastases

- CA-125: >35 units/mL
- Histopathology: Infiltrative destructive growth best demonstrated by clusters of disorganized cells, usually with desmoplasia
- PET scan or integrated PET-CT: High SUV uptake in abnormal lesions

Treatment

- **Early:** stage IA/IB or grade 1 or 2: comprehensive surgical staging
- **Early:** stage IC or IA/IB grade 3 disease: combination surgery, operative staging, and chemotherapy
- **Advanced:** stage II, III, and IV (completely or optimally debulked): intravenous and intra-peritoneal chemotherapy
- **Advanced:** stage II, III, or IV (suboptimally debulked): intravenous chemotherapy

Uterine Prolapse

Presentation

- Patients have a feeling of heaviness, fullness, or "falling out" in the perineal area.
- Low uterus: Cervix may be seen protruding from the introitus
- Total Descensus: Patient is aware that a mass has actually prolapsed out of the introitus. The patient may report pain or vaginal bleeding due to ulceration or damage.
- There is often discharge from the cervix and vagina when secondary infection occurs

Evaluation

- A prolapse into the upper barrel of the vagina is called *first degree*
- A prolapse through the vaginal barrel to the region of the introitus, it is *second degree*
- If cervix and uterus prolapse out through the introitus, it is called *third degree* or *total*
- In total prolapse the vagina is everted around the uterus and cervix and completely exteriorized
- Patient in danger of developing dryness, thickening, and chronic inflammation of the vaginal epithelium

Management

- Medical management of such conditions involves the use of a pessary
- Smith-Hodge, donut, cube, or inflatable
- If the patient is a young woman and pregnant, it is important to replace the uterus before it enlarges and becomes trapped in the lower pelvis or vagina
  - Edema may cause incarceration and even loss of blood supply to the uterus
- In a postmenopausal woman, estrogen replacement for at least 30 days with vaginal estrogen cream may help improve the vitality of the vaginal epithelium, the cervix, and the vasculature of these organs

- Operative repair for prolapse of the uterus and cervix generally involves a vaginal hysterectomy with a vaginal vault suspension

Folic Acid in Pregnancy

- 1-5mg of folic acid (300mg in PNV)
- Folic acid helps prevent neural tube defects
- Serious birth defects of the spinal cord (Spinal bifida) and the brain (Anencephaly). Neural tube defects occur at a very early stage of development, before many women even know they're pregnant.

Alpha-Fetoprotein

Not reliable test if past16-18wks prenatal

Alpha-fetoprotein screening: Check during weeks 16-18

- Should be decreased, checking for open neural tube defects, Trisomy 18 and 21 (will be increased in these diseases)

Glucose tolerance test

- This is indicated with an abnormal glucose challenge test (GCT) which is usually done at 24-28 weeks;
- If a patient has risk factors (age >25, previous macroscopic infant, previous unexplained fetal demise, previous pregnancy with GDM, family history, history of PCOS and/ or obesity)

- GCT is done in the first trimester, if negative then its repeated at weeks 24-28

Order of delivery and Naegele's Rule

Naegele's Rule: (*LMP - 3mo +1 week*)

Order of Delivery

- Contractions → dilation and effacement → crowning → deliver baby → hold baby on forearm → clamp and cut cord → dry baby and hand to parent

Calculate APGAR

- This score is given for each sign at *one minute* and *five minutes* after the birth. If there are problems with the baby an additional score is given *at 10 minutes*
- A score of 7-10 is considered normal
- 4-7 might require some resuscitative measures\
- *3 and below requires immediate resuscitation*

	Sign	0 Points	1 Point	2 Points
A	Activity (Muscle Tone)	Absent	Arms and Legs Flexed	Active Movement
P	Pulse	Absent	Below 100 bpm	Above 100 bpm
G	Grimace (Reflex Irritability)	No Response	Grimace	Sneeze, cough, pulls away
A	Appearance (Skin Color)	Blue-gray, pale all over	Normal, except for extremities	Normal over entire body
R	Respiration	Absent	Slow, irregular	Good, crying

Preeclampsia VS. Eclampsia

Presentation

Lowering of the effective presser dose of infused angiotensin II

- Abnormal weight gain and edema
- Elevated blood pressure
- Placental infarctions resulting in retroplacental hemorrhage or abruption
- Visual disturbances
- Increased reflex irritability or hyper reflexia

Evaluation

Increase in hematocrit

- Proteinuria
- Increase in serum uric acid concentrations
- *Thrombocytopenia MC*
- DIC

Management

Delivery is the ***only*** definitive cure

- Full maternal history and physical
- Careful fetal evaluation
- US
- Non-stress Test
- Hospitalization- rest and observation if stable

MgSO4 to prevent convulsions

Placenta Previa (painless bleed) vs. Abruptio (painful bleed)

Abruptio placenta

Presentation

- *Painful vaginal bleeding*
- Uterine tenderness
- Hyperactivity
- Increased uterine tone
- Abdominal pain
- Fetal distress
- Fetal demise

Evaluation

- Clinical dx
- US may detect only 2%

Management

- Careful maternal hemodynamic and fetal monitoring
- Serial evaluation of hematocrit and coagulation profile
- Delivery
- Blood products should be available
- Tocolytics or uterine relaxants are contraindicated

Placenta Previa

Presentation

- Intermittent painless vaginal bleeding

Evaluation

- US- Transabdominal US has an accuracy of 95%
- Transvaginal US can accurately dx is virtually all cases

Management

- Excessive bleeding: C-section
    - No profuse bleeding: expectant therapy in hospital on bed rest
    - 36 weeks if lungs are mature: C-section

Postpartum hemorrhage is the #1 cause uterine Atony

Drugs that are safe to use in pregnancy and breastfeeding vs. those that are not safe

Most vulnerable stage is from *day 17 to day 56 post-conception* (or day 31 to day 71 by gestational age)

Safe

- Fluoxetine (Antianaxiety)
- Heparin
- Chlorpromazine, Haloperidol (Antipsychotics, BF)

- Acetaminophen (BF)
- Meperidine (Narcotic, BF)
- Digoxin (BF)
- Methyldopa, Propanolol (HTN, BF)

Not Safe

- Alcohol
- Meprobamate, Chlordiazepoxide (Antianxiety)
- Aminopterin, Methotrexate (Antineoplastic)
- Busulfan, Chlorambucil, Cyclophosphamide, Nitrogen Mustard (Alkylating Agents)
- Warfarin
- Dilantin
- Trimethadone, Paramethadone, Oxazolidinedione anticonvulsants
- Carbamazepine, Valparoic Acid
- Phenobarbital
- Estrogen-progestin combos
- DES
- Isotretinoin, Etretinate (Retinoids)
- Tobacco, Illicit Drugs
- Infectious Agents
- Radiation

Chapter Eight

Surgery, Suturing & Knot Tying

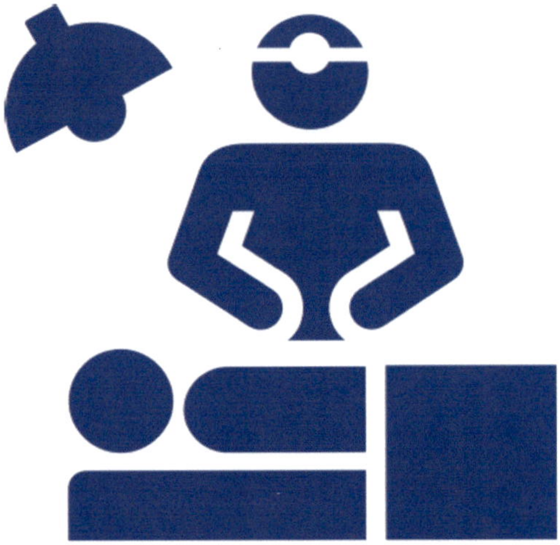

Compartment Syndrome: 5 P's

- Pain
- Pallor
- Pulseless
- Paresthesias
- Pressure (increased)

Pancreatitis Risk Factors

- Alcohol abuse: 2 for men/ day, 1 for women/ day
- Family history:
- Gull stones: MCC of acute pancreatitis
- CF: deficient pancreatic enzymes
- Smoking
- Meds such as Abx and Estrogen
- High Triglycerides: MC >500

Anal cancer

- Bleeding from the anus or rectum
- Pain in the area of the anus
- A mass or growth in the anal canal
- Anal itching

Colicky pain

- Pain, which starts and stops abruptly
- It occurs due to muscular contractions of a hollow tube (colon, ureter, gall bladder, etc.) in attempt to relieve the obstruction by forcing content out

Esophageal Variceal Bleed

- Band Ligation is the most effective treatment
- Clotting medicine injection, place a rubber band around the bleeding veins.
- The procedure is done using an endoscope.
- A medication that vasoconstricts may be used such as *octreotide or vasopressin*.
- Rarely, a tube is put into the stomach and inflated with air. This produces pressure against the bleeding veins (balloon tamponade).

Coffee Ground Emesis

- MC: (*Upper GI Bleed*)
- Liver disease like alcoholic liver disease, cirrhosis, or liver cancer
- Cancer of esophagus, pancreas, or stomach
- Peptic or stomach ulcers
- Bleeding esophageal varices or enlarged veins in the esophagus
- Diseases such as the Ebola virus, hemophilia B, or yellow fever
- Gastritis or inflammation of the stomach
- Gastroesophageal reflux disease (GERD)
- Glomerulonephritis (a type of kidney disease)
- Aspirin overdose

Grave's disease (Hyperthyroidism)

- First line Treatment is radioactive iodine
- Anti-thyroid medication- Methimazole
- Beta Blockers
- Opthalmopathy:
  Corticosteroids
  Decompression surgery

5 W's of post op fever

Day 1	Wind	atelectasis, pneumonia, and aspiration
Day 3	Water	UTI/ Phlebitis from IV
Day 5	Wound	wound infection
Day 7	Walking	DVT/PE
Day 7+	Wonder Drugs	drug induced by something we gave

(-) DRE, asymptomatic patient and an elevated PSA

- PSA is a serine protease and is increased in prostate cancer. PSA >4ng/mL is considered abnormal. PSA > 20ng/mL or PSA > 10ng/mL is associated with increased risk of metastatic disease. In such cases a bone scan and pelvic CT scan should be performed
- Men with abnormal PSA values can *repeat the PSA several weeks later*, particularly for borderline elevations below 7.0 ng/mL.
- Primary care providers should refer men with a PSA level above 7 ng/mL without further testing; a specialist can decide whether to

proceed directly to biopsy or perform additional testing

- Before any retest, *men should abstain from ejaculation and bike riding for at least 48 hours*

Antibiotics Induced Colitis

- C Diff- MC from (Clindamycin)

Electrolyte imbalances

Hypernatremia

DDx

- Inadequate hydration, diarrhea, vomiting, diabetes insipidus, tachypnea, Hyperaldosteronism, osmotic diuresis (urea or glucose)

- If inpatient, think iatrogenic! Inappropriate IV

Lab Study

- BMP

Treatment

- D5W, ¼ NS, or ½ NS

Hyponatremia

DDx

- Too much water compared to sodium (ex. Water intake without excretion, inability to suppress ADH)
- If inpatient, think iatrogenic! fluid excess MC
- Cardiac, renal failure, diarrhea, vomiting, SIADH

Lab Study

- BMP

Treatment

- If healthy renal function and mild to moderately severe symptoms, the serum sodium level may correct spontaneously.
- May use diuretics if patient is hypervolemic
- Patients with seizures, severe confusion, coma, or signs of brainstem

herniation should receive hypertonic (3%) saline

- Increase the serum sodium level by 4-6 mEq/L over the first 1-2 hours and *do not exceed 9mEq/L/Hr* or the patient may get pontine myelinosis

Hypercalcemia

DDx

- **Hyperparathyroidism- MC, malignancies, metastatic disease, ectopic PTH production, Vitamin D intoxication

Lab Study

- BMP

Treatment

- Isotonic NS with simultaneous administration of loop diuretics (NOT thiazides)

Hypocalcemia

Symptoms

- Tingling and numbness in extremities

DDx

- **Hypoalbuminemia- MC, hypoparathyroidism, vitamin D deficiency, malabsorption syndromes, acute pancreatitis, renal failure, short bowel syndrome, intestinal bypass, sepsis, diuretics, hypomagnesemia, rhabdomyolysis

Lab Study

- BMP

Treatment

- Acute: IV Calcium Gluconate or CaCl
- Chronic: Calcium or Vitamin D supplements

Hyperkalemia

- Small changes in serum K+: Major changes in body- 95% intracellular

DDx

- **Hemolysis- pseudohyperkalemia (get second blood sample)
- Iatrogenic overdose, blood transfusion, tissue trauma (hemolysis), renal failure, metabolic acidosis

Lab Study

- BMP

Treatment

- Urgent: IV Calcium (cardioprotective), EKG monitoring, Sodium bicarbonate IV
- Glucose & insulin

Non-urgent

- Furosemide

Severe cases require hemodialysis, which is the most rapid method of removing potassium from the body

Hypokalemia

DDx

- Diuretics, diet/IV, vomiting, diarrhea, sweating, metabolic alkalosis, dialysis

Lab Study

- BMP

Treatment

- Oral or IV KCl

Fun Fact:

- Hypokalemia is the most common electrolyte-mediated ileus in the surgical patient

Hypomagnesemia

DDx

- Low dietary intake (seen in TPN, elderly, malnourished, and with alcoholism), GI disorders such as Crohn's, hypoparathyroidism (hypocalcemia), long-term diuretic use, prolonged diarrhea, post-surgery, severe burns, renal failure

- Cause of unexplained cardiac arrhythmias & neuromuscular disorders
- Since a low magnesium level can cause persistently low calcium and potassium levels, it may help diagnose problems with calcium, potassium, phosphorus, and/or parathyroid hormone
  - If low Mg+ & low K+, you must fix low Mg+ b/c hypomagnesemia may make it impossible to correct hypokalemia

Lab Study

- Mg Level

Treatment

- Acute: MgSO4 IV

Chronic

- Magnesium Oxide PO

Crohn's vs. UC

	CROHNs	ULCERATIVE COLITIS
Origin	Terminal Ileum	Rectum
Progression	"Skip" lesions	Continuous
Thickness of Inflammation	Transmural	Sub-mucosa or mucosa
Symptoms	Crampy abdominal pain	Bloody Diarrhea
Complications	Fistulas, abscess, obstruction	Hemorrhage, toxic megacolon
X-Ray	String sign on barium X-ray	"Lead pipe"
Colon CA risk	Slight increase	Marked increase
Surgery	For strictures	Curative

ERCP vs. HIDA Scans

ERCP

Cholangiopancreatography

- This allows the common bile duct can be cannulated and a cholangiogram performed using fluoroscopy

Advantages

- Direct visualization of the biliary and pancreatic ducts, with the possibility of therapeutic intervention
- Mostly needed for stones in the common bile duct, in particular, when associated with obstructive jaundice, cholangitis, or gallstone pancreatitis
- ERCP is the diagnostic and often therapeutic procedure of choice.
- Once the endoscopic cholangiogram has shown ductal stones, sphincterotomy and stone extraction can be performed, and the common bile duct cleared of stones

HIDA

Biliary Radionuclide Scanning

- A noninvasive evaluation of the liver, gallbladder, bile ducts, and duodenum with both anatomic and functional information
- HIDA dye is injected intravenously, cleared by the Kupffer cells in the liver, and excreted in the bile
- Uptake by the liver is detected within 10 minutes, and the gallbladder, the bile ducts, and the duodenum are visualized within 60 minutes in fasting subjects
- MC used to diagnose acute cholecystitis
- Evidence of *cystic duct obstruction* on biliary scintigraphy is highly diagnostic for acute cholecystitis
- The sensitivity and specificity for the diagnosis are about 95%

Choledocolithiasis

- This is the presence of Gallstones in the gallbladder

Tetralogy of Fallot

4 Defects

Ventricular septal defect (VSD)

- Allows deoxygenated blood to flow into the aorta

Overriding large ascending aorta

- Lies just over the VSD, allowing the deoxygenated blood out

Right ventricular outflow obstruction

- AKA: Pulmonary stenosis
- Requires a valve change

Right ventricular hypertrophy

- R → L shunt
- Cyanotic defect

MC type of Cyanotic congenital heart defect

Pulmonary Embolism Findings

Clinical PE evidence of longstanding cyanotic defects

- Clubbing
- Polycythemia
- Paradoxical embolism
- Rt. sided emboli bypass the lungs and enter into the arterial circulation

MC Clinical Manifestations of Stroke

Broca's

- Frontal lobe: MCA- speech production deficit

Wernicke's

- Fluent aphasia: fluently connects words, lack meaning
- Non-Fluent aphasia: Use meaningful words in a non-fluent manner

Transient Ischemia Attacks

- Transient (<24 hours) focal symptoms and neurological deficits secondary to ischemia. Most resolve within 60 minutes (majority within 15 minutes)

Amaurosis fugax

- "Fleeting blindness" is a specific type of TIA characterized by transient monocular visual loss: caused by alteration of blood flow in

- the ophthalmic artery
- About 10% of pts with a TIA will have a stroke within the next 3 months and about 5% will have a stroke in the next 48 hours!
- 25-50% of large vessel atherothrombotic strokes are preceded by a TIA

Treatment

- For acute ischemic stroke, the recommendations initiating antihypertensive therapy only if blood pressure is higher than 220/120 mm Hg or if mean arterial pressure exceeds 130 mm Hg.

Noncardioembolic transient ischemic attack

- Antiplatelet agents, rather than oral anticoagulants, are recommended as initial therapy
- Aspirin 50-325 mg/day, a combination of aspirin and extended-release dipyridamole, and clopidogrel are all first-line options (class I recommendation)

Cardioembolic transient ischemic attack

- In patients who have atrial fibrillation in association with a TIA, long-term anticoagulation with warfarin to a target international normalized ratio (INR) of 2-3 is typically recommended
- Aspirin 325 mg/day is recommended for patients unable to take oral anticoagulants

Pneumothorax

Definition

This is a collapse of a lung that can cause respiratory compromise and can lead to death

Signs and Symptoms

- Acute pleuritic CP, dyspnea, tachypnea, tachycardia, decreased breath sounds on affected side, hyperresonance to percussion, decreased tactile fremitus, +/- respiratory distress
- Tension
  - Hypotension, absent breath sounds, distended jugular veins, tracheal

deviation, diaphoresis, cyanosis, cardiovascular collapse

Diagnosis

- CXR: presence of thin radiolucent pleural line, absence of vascular lung markings peripheral to the pleural line, tracheal deviation to opposite side of pneumothorax (tension)
- ECG: Tachycardia, nonspecific ST-segment changes, T wave inversion
- ABG: Hypoxia, normal PCO2

Thyroid Cancer

Papillary: Surgery (MC 80% less aggressive)

- MC in young adults
- 10 year survival 95%

Risk Factors

- Radiation at a young age, Gardner syndrome,
- 1/ mets to cervical lymph nodes
- Slow growing, painless mass

Treatment

- If small and no hx of rx to the neck: lobectomy, near total thyroidectomy, or total
- Post op need thyroid hormone, repeat iodine uptake study

Follicular: Surgery *TOTAL* thyroidectomy

- MC older adults (40-50yo females) comprises 10% thyroid cancers
- 10 year survival 65%
- RAS oncogene mutation
- Mets: bone (MC), liver, lung (spread though the blood)
- Well differentiated, rubbery, encapsulated

Cold and Hot Thyroid Nodules

Radionuclide Scans

- Cold-CANCER, Hypo function- *MC Papillary*
- Hot -Hyper function

Hassel Bach's triangle

Borders	Anatomy
Superior	Inferior Epigastric Vessels
Inferior	Inguinal Ligament
Medial	Rectus Abdominis Muscle

Rovsing Sign

- Palpation of the left lower quadrant of the abdomen
- Increase pain in the right lower quadrant if patient has a positive Rovsing's sign and may have appendicitis

Strangulated hernia

- Always an emergency surgery d/t compromised blood flow that could cause ischemia of the tissues

MC Location of Colon Cancer

- The most common colon cancer is *adenocarcinoma*.
- The most common site of colorectal cancer is the **sigmoid colon (25%)** followed by the rectum (21%) followed by cecum (20%)

Appendicitis

Etiology

- Blockage by fecalith, foreign body or tumor

Symptoms

- First symptom may be pain around belly button, may have nausea, vomiting, low fever.
- Pain moves to right lower abdomen and focuses at McBurney's point 12-48 hours after illness starts

Lab findings

- CBC may show increased leukocytes. Rise in CRP. Neither are specific

X-ray

- Feces in appendix.

- Abdominal CT most frequently used in adults to visualize lack of contrast in appendix, enlargement of appendix, appendiceal wall enhancement with contrast.
- Ultrasound: good in children to note fluid collection in right iliac fossa and visible appendix without blood flow

Treatment

- Appendectomy

SBO (Small Bowel Obstruction)

Symptoms

- Proximal: Colicky with bilious vomiting, less distention
- Distal: Long lasting pain that is progressive in nature and accompanied with distention

Early: diarrhea, hyperactive tinkly bowel sounds

Late: Constipation, Fever and tachycardia may be associated with strangulation.

- Changes in pain may indicate more serious complications such as an ischemic or strangulated bowel. Hypoactive bowel sounds

Etiology

- MC postsurgical adhesions, incarcerated groin hernias or other hernias, malignant tumor, IBD, volvulus

Surgical indications

- Strangulated obstruction is a surgical emergency, simple complete obstruction when non-operative trials fail

Prothrombin Time

Prothrombin time is a blood test that measures the time it takes for the plasma portion of your blood to clot

- Extrinsic pathway

- Factors I, II, VII, X (Factor VII most important)

With Warfarin: INR goal (2-3)

W/O warfarin: 11-13.5 seconds or INR (0.8-1.1)

Breast cancer

Inflammatory carcinoma

- Systemic chemo to shrink, then surgery, then radiation

Treatment

- Most commonly show HER2 gene: so response to Herceptin (Trastuzumad)
- Positive or negative sentinel nodes
    - (+) Axillary node dissection
    - (-) No dissection

Presentation

- Edema, Redness, "Peau d'orange", swollen lymph nodes, *bloody nipple discharge*
- Rapid onset, <6months, erythema over 1/3 of breast and + breast biopsy for invasive carcinoma

Breast Drainage

Pathologic discharge

- *Unilateral* from a single duct, **spontaneously**, and persistent
- Serosanginous, serous, or clear is associated with an increased risk of malignancy

Imaging

- MRI or ductogram: Contrast is injected into the breast duct with US/ guidance

Treatment

- If pathological discharge is ruled out then a terminal duct excision (surgical excision) is needed

Watery, Serous, Serosanguinous, and Bloody Discharges

- MCC: *Intraductal Papillomas*
- Fibrocystic disease, advanced duct ectasia, cancer of the breast, and vascular engorgement in near-term pregnancy can also be causative

Hemorrhoids

Painful swollen veins in the lower portion of the rectum or anus

Dentate line

- Determines between *Internal* and *External*

Flexible Sigmoidoscopy and Colonoscopy

- Best evaluation modality generally in a retroflexed view

Obstruction Small and Large Bowel

SB: *MC postsurgical adhesions*

- Dilated loops of small bowel proximal to the obstruction
- Predominantly central dilated loops
- Three instances of dilatation over 3 cm
- Valvulae conniventes are visible
- There may be fluid levels if the study is erect (non-standard technique)

Also, the *string-of-beads sign*: small pockets of gas within a fluid-filled small bowl

LB: *60% malignancies*, 20% diverticular disease, 5% volvulus

- In age group > 60
- Radiological findings- colonic distension: gaseous secondary to gas-producing organisms in faeces
- Collapsed distal colon
- Small bowel dilatation, depends on
  - Duration of obstruction and incompetence of the Ileocaecal valve

Hypovolemic Shock

- A life-threatening condition that results when you lose more than 20 percent (one-fifth) of your body's blood or fluid supply
- This severe fluid loss makes it impossible for the heart to pump sufficient blood to your body

The sign of *external* hemorrhaging is bleeding profusely at the site of injury

Signs of *internal* hemorrhaging

- Abdominal pain
- Blood in the stool
- Blood in the urine
- Vaginal bleeding (heavy, usually outside of normal menstruation)
- Vomiting blood
- Chest pain
- Abdominal swelling

MC causes of pancreatitis

- **Alcohol Pancreatitis, Cholelithiasis**
- Adenocarcinoma involving the head of the pancreas the ampulla of Vater, the distal common bile duct (CBD) and the duodenum are considered together because they are indistinguishable clinically
- ***75% of pancreatic adenocarcinomas are in the head of the pancreas***, while 25% are in the rest of the body or tail

Cholangitis

- Ascending (caused by gall stones) can be life threatening!

This is an infection (*MC Bacterial*) of the common bile duct,

- Bile is a liquid made by the liver that helps digest food.
- MC: Anaerobic organisms such as Clostridium and Bacteroides

Risk factors

- History of gallstones, Sclerosing cholangitis, HIV, narrowing of the common bile duct, and, rarely, travels to countries where you might get a parasite infection

Hernias

Surgical emergency if strangulated

- **Femoral:** MC in Women- MC to involve bowel
- **Inguinal:** 75% of abdominal wall hernias
- **Indirect: MC** hernia in (men and women of any age). Indirect may protrude into scrotum
- **Direct:** MC in older people

Gallstones

Treatment: Cholecystectomy

MC component of stone in US

- MC, Stones made of *cholesterol*. *Cholesterol gallstones are not related to cholesterol levels in the blood*

Choledocholithiasis

This is the presence of gallstones in the common bile duct. This condition causes jaundice and liver cell damage, and requires treatment by cholecystectomy and/or ERCP

Symptoms

- Very similar to acute cholecystitis

Physical exam

- Cutaneous and scleral icterus, charcot triad, may be asymptomatic or have RUQ pain with rebound and guarding, murphy's sign, fever

Diagnostic radiologic studies

- Endoscopic retrograde, CBC: elevated WBC count may indicate or raise suspicion of cholecystitis

Colonoscopy/Barium Swallow Contraindication

(When perforation)

Administration of colloids for a burn

(After 24 hr)

Carpal Tunnel Syndrome

Treatment

- Splinting, analgesics and rest
- Procedure includes division of the flexor retinaculum when unresponsive to splinting

Carpal Tunnel in Pregnancy

- The fluid retention and swelling that's so common during pregnancy can increase the pressure in this relatively narrow and inflexible space, compressing the median nerve that runs through it

Nerve: Median

Treatment of Cutaneous Abscess

- I&D abscess, *irrigate* with peroxide and then treat with broad spectrum Abx until culture is read and organism is identified
- Irrigation with water is the single most important action to prevent infection

Suturing

1. **Simple Interrupted**
   Indications: (MC Stitch)
   Use "Rule of Halves"
   Depth of needle penetrations is determined by wound depth to ensure no dead space.
   "Bites" on each side of the wound should be symmetrical (wide as wound is deep)

2. **Vertical Mattress**
   Indications: (2nd MC Stitch)
   Used for closing deeper wounds to eliminate the dead space
   Far-Far, Near-Near

3. **Horizontal Mattress**
   Indications:
   Used when there is a flap of tissue or tension of the stitch is on the one side (vascular and avascular wound)
   Stitch looks like a box
   Good for spreading out tension in frail skin

1-3 https://www.youtube.com/watch?v=qGU4Pn4UnME

4. **Running Suture**
   Indications:
   Can be performed quickly and applied tightly if "locked"
   Railroad tracks
   https://www.youtube.com/watch?v=ODZtJL_gb4E

5. **Subcuticular**
   Indications:
   No suture is visible after procedure
   Does not need to be removed (absorbed)
   Start at 3:58
   https://www.youtube.com/watch?v=iYts9c6Jrx8

Knot Tying

1. **One- Handed – 3 finger, Thumb**
   https://www.youtube.com/watch?v=HTxT60u2Lj0
2. **Two-Handed- Gun, Triangle**
   https://www.youtube.com/watch?v=_lvQ2YJ0RjQ
3. **Instrument**
   https://www.youtube.com/watch?v=-smZKFnC-U8

Chapter Nine

Pharmacology / ABX

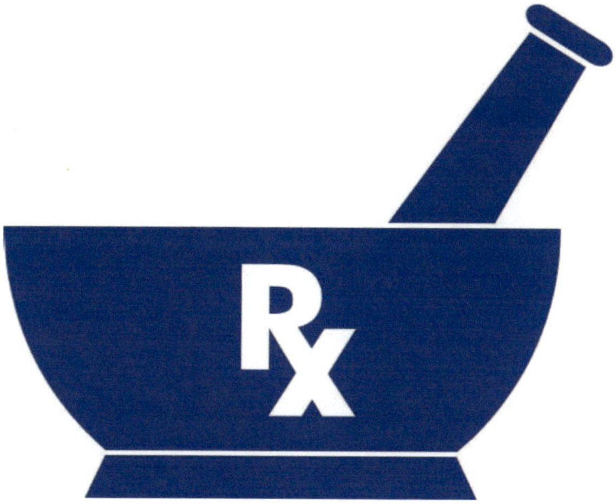

COMMON MEDICATIONS

Oral Anti-MSSA ABX

Gold standard = dicloxacillin

- Silver standard = cephalexin
- Doxycycline, TMP-SMX, clindamycin also effective (use if allergic to β-lactam)
- Note: MSSA = methicillin-susceptible S. aureus

Parenteral Anti-MSSA ABX

Gold standard = nafcillin

- Silver standard = cefazolin
- Bronze standard = vancomycin
- Note: MSSA = methicillin-susceptible S. aureus

Oral Anti-MRSA ABX

- **Linezolid & Tedizolid**
- Doxycycline & Minocycline
    - TMP-SMX
- Clindamycin
- Note: MRSA = Methicillin-resistant S. aureus

Parenteral Anti-MRSA

- **"Gold standard" = vancomycin**
- Other options
- Linezolid & Tedizolid
- Daptomycin
- Tigecycline
- Telavancin, Dalbavancin, & Oritavancin
    - Ceftaroline

Oral Anti-**Pseudomonal** ABX

- **Ciprofloxacin & levofloxacin**

Parenteral Anti-**Pseudomonal** ABX

- **Piperacillin/tazobactam**
- Aztreonam
- Ceftazidime or cefepime
- Ciprofloxicin or levofloxacin
  - Tobramycin
- Doripenem > Meropenem > Imipenem
  - Not ertapenem

Oral Anti-**VRE** ABX

- **Linezolid & tedizolid**
- Note: VRE = Vancomycin-resistant enterococcus

Parenteral Anti-**VRE** ABX

- **Linezolid**
- Daptomycin
- Tigecycline
- Telavancin, Dalbavancin, & Oritavancin

Oral Anti-**Anaerobic** ABX

- **Gold standard = metronidazole or amoxicillin /**
- **clavulanate**
- Silver standard = clindamycin

Parenteral Anti-Anaerobic ABX

- **Gold standard = β-lactam / β-lactamase inhibitor combo (ex. piperacillin/tazobactum)**
- Carbapenems (ex. imipenem)
- Metronidazole
- Silver standard = clindamycin
- Bronze standard = cephamycins (ex. cefoxitin)

Chapter Ten

Antibodies

Disease	Antibody
Addison's	Anti-CYP21A2 (p450-c21) or 21-hydroxylase, Anti- CYP11A1 and Anti-CYP17
Polymyositis/ Dermatomyositis	Antinuclear Ab (ANA), Anti-Ribonucleoprotein (RNP) Ab, Myositis specific Ab (Anti-Jo-1 Ab, Anti-Mi-2 Ab, Anti-PM Sci Ab and Anti-Ku Ab)
Monoclonal Gammopathy	Anti-Mag Ab
Cryoglobulinemia	Anti- HCV Ab
Systemic Lupus Erythematosus (SLE)	ANA, Anti-Ro, Anti- La, Anti-Sm Ab, Anti-double stranded DNA Ab
Rheumatoid Arthritis	IgM rheumatoid factor, Ab against Fe portion of IgG
Factor VIII Deficiency	Anti-factor VIII Ab
Peripheral Neuropathy	Anti-MAG Ab, IgM Anti-glycoconjugate Ab
IgM Polyneuropathy	Anti-Myelin Associated Glycoprotein (MAG) Ab
Chronic Neuropathy	IgM Anti-ganglioside Ab
Hashimoto's Thyroiditis	Anti TPO Ab, Anti TG Ab, Anti-Thyroid Stimulating Hormone Receptor (TSHR) Ab
Anti-phospholipid Ab Syndrome	Antiphospholipid Ab
Multiple Sclerosis	Anti-Myelin Basic Protein, Anti-Myelin Oligodendrocytic glycoprotein Ab
Drug Induced SLE	Anti- Histone Ab
Sub-acute Cutaneous SLE	SSA (RO) Ab
Scleroderma	Anti-Scl- 70 Ab
CREST	Anti-Centromere Ab

Disease	**Antibody**
Sjogren's	SSA (RO) and SSB (LA) Ab
Wegener's Granulamatosis	C-ANCA
Polyarteritis Angitis	P-ANCA
Celiac Disease	Anti-tissue Transglutamase Ab, Anti-endomysial Ab
Primary Biliary Cirrhosis	Anti-mitochondrial Ab
Guillian-Barre Syndrome	Cross reactive Ab to GM1 ganglioside Ab or GQ1b ganglioside
Myasthenia Gravis	Anti- AcH Receptor Ab (AChR)
Giant Cell Arteritis	Serum Anti- endothelial cell Ab
Kawasaki's Disease	Anti- endothelial Ab, ANCA

Chapter Eleven

Muscles and Functions

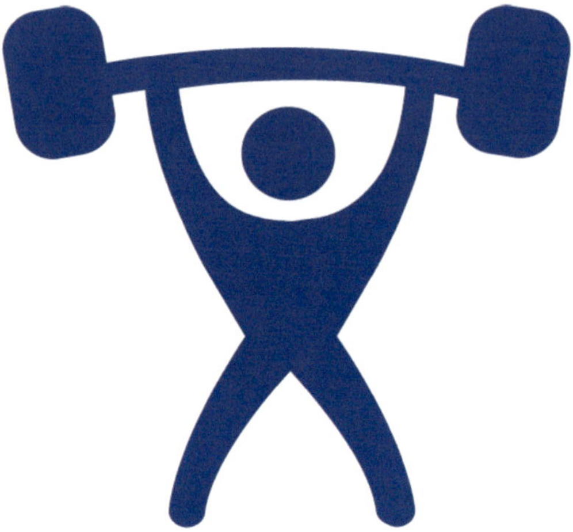

MUSCLES OF THE UPPER EXTREMITY				
Muscle	**Attachment**	**Attachment**	**Innervation**	**Function**
Pectoralis Major	anterior medial 1/2 clavicle & anterior sternum	greater tubercle	medial & lateral pec nerves	Adduction and medial rotation
Pectoralis Minor	ribs 3-5 at costal cartilage	medial superior coracoid process	medial pectoral nerve	draws scap. Ant & infer
Subclavius	Jxn rib 1 & costal cartilage	middle inferior 1/3 clavicle	subclavian nerve	clavicular depression
Serratus Anterior	lateral external ribs 1-8	anterior medial border of scapula	long thoracic nerve	scapular protraction
Trapezius	external occipital protuberance, spinal processes C7-T12	lateral 1/3 of scap, spine, acromion	spinal accessory nerve (cranial nerve XI)	scap elev, depress, retraction
Latissimus Dorsi	processes T7-sacrum, iliac crest	Intertubercu-lar groove	thoracodorsal nerve	extension, adduction, medial rotation
Levator Scapulae	Transverse processes C1-C4	Medial Superior Scapula	Dorsal Scapular Nerve	Elevates Scapula
Rhomboid Minor	Medial scapular border (superior to major)	Spinous Processes C7-T1	Dorsal Scapular Nerve	scapular retraction
Rhomboid Major	Medial scapular border (inferior to minor)	Spinous Processes T2-T5	Dorsal Scapular Nerve	scapular retraction

Muscle	Attachment	Attachment	Innervation	Function
Deltoid	lateral 1/3 of clavicle, spine, acromion	deltiod tuberosity	axillary nerve	flexion, abduction, extension
Supraspinatus	supraspinatus fossa	superior facet of greater tubercle	suprascapular nerve	abduction to 30'
Infraspinatus	infraspinatus fossa	middle facet of greater tubercle	suprascapular nerve	external rotation of hum.
Teres Minor	middle lateral scapular border	inferior facet of greater tubercle	axillary nerve	external rotation of hum.
Teres Major	inferior angle of scapula	Medial lip of intertubercular groove	Lower Subscapular Nerve	Adduction and Medial Rotation
Subscapularis	subscapular fossa	Lesser tubercle	upper & lower subscap. Nerves	medial rotation
Biceps Brachii	Long Head:supra-glenoid tubercle Short Head: coracoid process	Tuberosity of the Radius	Musculocutaneous nerve	flexion, supination
Brachialis	distal 1/2 anterior humerus	coronoid process, ulnar tuberosity	Musculocutaneous nerve	elbow flexion
Coracobrachialis	tip of coracoid process	middle medial 1/3 humerus	Musculocutaneous nerve	flexion, adduction
Triceps Brachii	infraglenoid tubercle, posterior humerus	proximal olecranon, forearm fascia	radial nerve	extension
Anconeus	lateral superior posterior ulna	lateral epicondyle	radial nerve	forearm extension, elbow stability

Muscle	Attachment	Attachment	Innervation	Function
Pronator Teres	coronoid process, medial epicondyle	middle lateral radius	Median Nerve	pronation, elbow flexion
Flexor Carpi Radialis	medial epicondyle	base of second and third metacarpal	Median Nerve	flexes, radial deviation
Palmaris Longus	medial epicondyle	aponeurosis and palmer retinaculum	Median Nerve	tightens aponeurosis, wrist flexion
Flexor Carpi Ulnaris	medial epicondyle, olecranon process	pisiform, hamate hook, 5th metacarpal	ulnar nerve	hand flexion, ulnar deviation
Flexor Digitorum Superficialis	medial epicondyle, superior anterior radius	middle anterior phalanges 2-5	Median Nerve	PIP, MCP Flexion
Flexor Digitorum Profundus	proximal, medial, anterior ulna	distal phalanges 2-5	1/2 median, 1/2 ulnar	DIP Flexion
Flexor Pollicis Longus	anterior radius, interosseus membrane	base distal phalanx of thumb	Median Nerve	thumb flexion
Pronator Quadratus	distal anterior ulna	distal anterior 1/4 radius	Median Nerve	pronation, binds ulna and radius
Brachio-radialis	lateral supracondylar ridge of hum.	lateral distal end of radius proximal to styloid process	radial nerve	forearm flexion
Extensor Carpi Radialis Longus	lateral supracondylar ridge	dorsal base of 2nd metacarpal	radial nerve	hand extension, radial deviation
Extensor Carpi Radialis Brevis	lateral epicondyle	dorsal base of 3rd metacarpal	radial nerve	hand extension, radial deviation

Muscle	Attachment	Attachment	Innervation	Function
Extensor Digitorum	lateral epicondyle	extensor expansion digits 2-5	radial nerve	extends MCP, IP joints
Extensor Digiti Minimi	lateral epicondyle	base of proximal phalanx of 5th finger	radial nerve	extends 5th finger
Extensor Carpi Ulnaris	lateral epicondyle	base of dorsal aspect of 5th metacarpal	radial nerve	hand extension, ulnar deviation
Supinator	lateral epicondyle, radial collateral ligament, annular ligament, supinator fossa, ulnar crest	proximal posterior radius	radial nerve	supination
Abductor Pollicis Longus	posterior ulna and radius, inteross. Membrane	base of 1st metacarpal	radial nerve	thumb abduction and extension
Extensor Pollicis Brevis	posterior distal radius, inteross. Membrane	base of proximal phalanx of thumb	radial nerve	extends MCP, CMC joints of thumb
Extensor Pollicis Longus	posterior ulna and inteross. Membrane	base of distal phalanx of thumb	radial nerve	Extend IP, MCP, CMC joints of thumb
Extensor Indicis	posterior distal 1/3 of ulna, inteross. Membrane	base of proximal phalanx of 2nd finger	radial nerve	extends 2nd finger and wrist
Abductor Pollicis Brevis	scaphoid, trapezium, flexor retinaculum	base of proximal phalanx of first digit	Median Nerve	thumb abductor

Muscle	Attachment	Attachment	Innervation	Function
Flexor Pollicis Brevis	flexor retinaculum, trapezium, 1st metacarpal	base of proximal phalanx of first digit	Median Nerve	thumb flexion
Opponens Pollicis	flexor retinaculum, trapezium	first metacarpal	Median Nerve	opposes the thumb
Adductor Pollicis	ulnar side of the base phalanx of the thumb	capitate bone, base of 2-3 metacarpals	ulnar nerve	adducts the thumb
Abductor Digiti Minimi	pisiform, tendon of flexor carpi ulnaris	base of proximal phalanx of fifth finger	Ulnar Nerve	abducts the pinkie finger
Flexor Digiti Minimi Brevis	flexor retinaculum, hook of the hamate	base of proximal phalanx of fifth finger	Ulnar Nerve	flexes 5th MCP joint
Opponens Digiti Minimi	flexor retinaculum, hook of the hamate	5th metacarpal bone	Ulnar Nerve	Opposes pinkie finger
Lumbricals 1-2	FDP Tendon	digits 2-3	Median Nerve	extend IP, flexes MCP
Lumbricals 3-4	FDP Tendon	digits 4-5	Ulnar Nerve	extend IP, flexes MCP
Palmar Interossei 1-4	base of metacarpals 1, 2, 4, 5	base of corresponding proximal phalanx	Ulnar Nerve	adduct digits (PAD)
Dorsal Interossei 1-4	base of metacarpals. Two heads coming from adjacent sides	lateral proximal phalanx of 2-3, medial proximal phalanx of 4-5	Ulnar Nerve	abduct digits (DAB)

<table>
<tr><th colspan="6">MUSCLES OF THE LOWER EXTREMITY</th></tr>
<tr><th>Muscle</th><th>Attachment</th><th>Attachment</th><th>Function</th><th colspan="2">Innervation</th></tr>
<tr><td>Psoas minor</td><td>T12-L1</td><td>anterior ilium</td><td>Trunk Flexion</td><td colspan="2">Root L1</td></tr>
<tr><td>Psoas major</td><td>T12-L5</td><td>lesser trochanter (conjoint tendon)</td><td>Trunk AND Hip Flexion</td><td colspan="2">Roots L2-L3</td></tr>
<tr><td>Iliacus</td><td>iliac fossa</td><td>lesser trochanter (conjoint tendon)</td><td>hip flexion</td><td colspan="2">Femoral nerve</td></tr>
<tr><td>Gluteus maximus</td><td>sacrum, ilium</td><td>IT band</td><td>hip extension, abduction, lateral rotation</td><td colspan="2">inferior gluteal nerve</td></tr>
<tr><td>Gluteus medius</td><td>iliac crest</td><td>greater trochanter</td><td>abduction</td><td colspan="2">superior gluteal nerve</td></tr>
<tr><td>Gluteus minimus</td><td>gluteal lines of ilium</td><td>greater trochanter</td><td>abduction, medial rotation</td><td colspan="2">superior gluteal nerve</td></tr>
<tr><td>Piriformis</td><td>anterior sacrum</td><td>superior border of greater trochanter of the femur</td><td>lateral rotation and abduction</td><td>S1-S2</td><td rowspan="4">P
G
O
G
O
Q</td></tr>
<tr><td>Gemelli Superior</td><td>ischial spine</td><td>medial greater trochanter of femur</td><td>lateral rotation and abduction</td><td>Nerve to obturator internus</td></tr>
<tr><td>Obturator Internus</td><td>Obturator membrane surface</td><td>medial greater trochanter of femur</td><td>lateral rotation and abduction</td><td>L5 S1</td></tr>
<tr><td>Gemelli Inferior</td><td>ischial tuberosity</td><td>medial greater trochanter of femur</td><td>lateral rotation and abduction</td><td>Nerve to quatratus femoris</td></tr>
</table>

Muscle	Attachment	Attachment	Function	Innervation
Obturator Externus	obterator foramen margins and membrane	trochanteric fossa of femur	lateral rotation	obturator nerve
Quadratus Femoris	lateral ischial tuberosity	intertrochanteri c crest	lateral rotation	nerve to quadratus femoris L5 S1
Tensor Fascia lata	anterior iliac crest	IT Band, Gerdy's tubercle	Hip flexion, abduction	superior gluteal nerve
Sartorius	ASIS	anteromedial tibia via pes anserine tendon	Hip flexion, abduction, external rotation, knee flexion	femoral nerve
Rectus Femoris	AIIS	quadriceps tendon	knee and hip extension	femoral nerve
Vastus lateralis	greater trochanter, lateral lip of linea aspera	quadriceps tendon	knee extension	femoral nerve
Vastus medialis	intertrochanteric line and medial lip of linea aspera	quadriceps tendon	knee extension	femoral nerve
Vastus intermedius	anterior and lateral femur	quadriceps tendon	knee extension	femoral nerve
Biceps femoris	long head: ischial tuberosity, short head: linea aspera and lateral supracondylar line	lateral head of fibula, lateral condyle of tibia	extends hip and knee flexion	long head: tibial nerve, short head: common fibular nerve

Muscle	Attachment	Attachment	Function	Innervation
Semitend inosus	ischial tuberosity	medial superior tibia (pes anserine)	extend hip, flex knee, medial rotation	Tibial nerve
Semimem branosus	ischial tuberosity	posterior medial condyle of tibia	extend hip, flex knee, medial rotation	Tibial nerve
Gracilis	body and inferior ramus of pubis	superior medial tibia	adducts thigh, flexes legm medial rotation	obturator nerve
Pectineus	Superior Pubic Ramus	Lesser trochanter, linea aspera	adduction, medial rotation	femoral nerve
Adductor longus	body of pubis	middle third of linea aspera	adducts thigh	obturator nerve
Adductor brevis	body and inferior ramus of pubis	pectineal line, proximal linea aspera	adducts thigh	obturator nerve
Adductor Magnus	inferior pubic ramus, ramus of ischium, ischial tuberosity	gluteal tuberosity, linea aspera, adductor tubercle of femur	adducts and extends hip	obturator nerve and Tibial nerve
Gastrocn emius	lateral and medial femoral condyles	achilles tendon	plantar flexion, knee flexion	Tibial nerve
Soleus	superior-posterior tibia and fibula	achilles tendon	plantarflexion	Tibial nerve
Plantaris	lateral supracondylar ridge of femur	posterior calcaneus	plantar flexion, knee flexion	Tibial nerve

Muscle	Attachment	Attachment	Function	Innervation
Popliteus	lateral femoral condyle	posterior tibia	internal rotation of tibia	Tibial nerve
Tibialis Anterior	lateral condyle of tibia	medial cuneiform and base of 1st MT	dorsiflexion and inversion	deep fibular nerve
Extensor Digitorum Longus	lateral condyle of tibia, fibula and interosseous membrane	distal phalanges of lateral 4 digits	toe extension and dorsiflexion	deep fibular nerve
Extensor Hallucis Longus	middle anterior fibula and interosseus membrane	dorsal base of distal phalanx of great toe	1st toe extension and dorsiflexion	deep fibular nerve
Flexor hallucis longus	inferior posterior fibula	base of distal phalanx of great toe	great toe flexion	Tibial nerve
Flexor digitorum longus	medial posterior tibia	base distal phalanges of lateral 4 digits	flexes 4 lateral digits, plantarflexes ankle	Tibial nerve
Tibialis Posterior	interosseus membrane, posterior tibia and fibula	tuberosity of navicular, cuneiform, and cuboid	plantarflexion , inversion	Tibial nerve
Fibularis Longus	head and superior lateral fibula	base of 1st MT and medial ceneiform	plantarflexion , eversion	superficial fibular nerve
Fibularis Brevis	inferior two third of lateral fibula	Dorsal surface of tuberosity on lateral side of base of 5th MT	plantarflexion , eversion	superficial fibular nerve
Fibularis Tertius	inferior third of anterior fibula	dorsal base of 5th MT	dorsiflexion and eversion	deep fibular nerve

Muscle	Attachment	Attachment	Function	Innervation
Adductor hallucis	bases of MTs 2-4, plantar ligaments	lateral base proximal phalanx of 1st digit	adducts 1st digit	Lateral Plantar Nerve
Abductor digiti minimi	tuberocity of calcaneus	lateral side of base proximal phalanx of 5th digit	abducts fifth toe	Lateral Plantar Nerve
Quadratus plantae	med/lat calcaneus	tendon of FDL	Assists flexor digitorum longus	Lateral Plantar Nerve
Plantar interossei	bases, medial sides of MT 3-5	Base, medial sides of phalanges 3-5	Adduct digits 2-4, flex MTP joints	Lateral Plantar Nerve
Dorsal interossei	Adjacent sides of metatarsals 1-5	med, lateral sides of phalanges	abducts digits 2-4 and flexes MTP joints	Lateral Plantar Nerve
Lumbricals	tendons of FDL	dorsal surfaces of proximal phalanges	flexes proximal phalanges of 2-5 toes	Medial (1) and Lateral (3) Plantar Nerves
Abductor hallucis	medial tubercle of the calcaneus	medial base of proximal phalanx of 1st digit	abducts and flexes big toe	Medial Plantar Nerve
Flexor digitorum brevis	medial tubercle of the calcaneus	middle phalanges of lateral 4 digits	digit flexion	Medial Plantar Nerve
Flexor hallucis brevis	cuboid and lateral cuneiforms	base proximal phalanx of 1st digit	flexes proximal phalanx of 1st digit	Medial Plantar Nerve
Flexor digiti minimi brevis	Base of 5th MT	Base proximal phalanx of 5th digit	Flexes prox phalanx of 5th digit	Superficial Lateral Plantar Nerve

References

Tuberculosis:

Herchline, T., MD. (2015, October 22). Tuberculosis. Retrieved December 4, 2015, from http://emedicine.medscape.com/article/230802-overview

Suturing:

A. (2012). 3 Interrupted Sutures: Simple, Vertical Mattress, & Horizontal Mattress.mov. Retrieved April 22, 2016, from https://www.youtube.com/watch?v=qGU4Pn4UnME

Cholesterol:

ATP III At-A-Glance: Quick Desk Reference. (2001, May). Retrieved October 28, 2015, from http://www.nhlbi.nih.gov/health-pro/guidelines/current/cholesterol-guidelines/quick-desk-reference-html

Cerebral Palsy:

Abdel-Hamid, H., MD. (2015, December 23). Cerebral Palsy. Retrieved January 3, 2016, from http://emedicine.medscape.com/article/1179555-overview

Hypercalcemia:

Agraharkar, M., MD. (2015, June 23). Hypercalcemia. Retrieved March 4, 2016, from http://emedicine.medscape.com/article/240681-overview

Angina Pectoris:

Alaeddini, J., MD. (2015, November 23). Angina Pectoris. Retrieved December 4, 2015, from http://emedicine.medscape.com/article/150215-overview

Sexually Transmitted Diseases:

An Overview of Sexually Transmitted Diseases (STDs). (n.d.). Retrieved March 12, 2016, from http://www.webmd.com/sex-relationships/health-sex-std-overview

Alzheimer Disease:

Anderson, H., MD. (2016, January 22). Alzheimer Disease. Retrieved February 4, 2016, from http://emedicine.medscape.com/article/1134817-overview

Radial Mononeuropathy:

Anderson, W., DO. (n.d.). Radial Mononeuropathy. Retrieved March 17, 2016, from http://emedicine.medscape.com/article/1141674-overview

Chancroid:

Arsove, P., MD. (2014, October 30). Chancroid. Retrieved December 3, 2015, from http://emedicine.medscape.com/article/214737-overview

Carpal Tunnel Syndrome:

Ashworth, N., MbCHB. (2015, July 1). Carpal Tunnel Syndrome. Retrieved February 17, 2016, from http://emedicine.medscape.com/article/327330-overview

Acute Epistaxis:

Bamimore, O., MD. (n.d.). Acute Epistaxis. Retrieved March 12, 2016, from http://emedicine.medscape.com/article/764719-overview

Human Bites:

Barrett, J., MD. (2016, March 22). Human Bites. Retrieved March 28, 2016, from http://emedicine.medscape.com/article/218901-overview

Scabies:

Barry, M., MD. (2015, November 18). Scabies. Retrieved December 5, 2015, from http://emedicine.medscape.com/article/1109204-overview

Systemic Lupus Erythematosus:

Bartels, C., MD. (2015, September 25). Systemic Lupus Erythematosus (SLE). Retrieved November 4, 2015, from http://emedicine.medscape.com/article/332244-overview

Ulcerative Colitis:

Basson, M., MD. (2015, November 18). Ulcerative Colitis. Retrieved March 12, 2016, from http://emedicine.medscape.com/article/183084-overview

Subarachnoid Hemorrhage:

Becske, T., MD. (n.d.). Subarachnoid Hemorrhage. Retrieved March 13, 2016, from http://emedicine.medscape.com/article/1164341-overview

Bereavement:

Bereavement Publications, Inc - Living With Loss Magazine, Hope and Healing Cards and Booklets, CareNotes Licensed Dealer. (n.d.). Retrieved February 4, 2016, from http://www.bereavementmag.com/

Chronic Myelogenous Leukemia:

Besa, E., MD. (2016, April 14). Chronic Myelogenous Leukemia (CML). Retrieved April 19, 2016, from http://emedicine.medscape.com/article/199425-overview

Osteoporosis:

Bethel, M., MD. (2016, March 11). Osteoporosis. Retrieved March 14, 2016, from http://emedicine.medscape.com/article/330598-overview

Tetralogy of Fallot:

Bhimji, S., MD. (2015, December 6). Tetralogy of Fallot. Retrieved February 2, 2016, from http://emedicine.medscape.com/article/2035949-overview

Intussusception:

Blanko, F., MD. (2016, March 3). Intussusception. Retrieved March 8, 2016, from http://emedicine.medscape.com/article/930708-overview

Blood Disorders:

Blood Disorder Types, Symptoms, and Treatments. (n.d.). Retrieved November 15, 2015, from http://www.webmd.com/cancer/lymphoma/blood-disorder-types-and-treatment from http://emedicine.medscape.com/article/253513-overview

Fibromyalgia:

Boomershine, C., MD. (2015, October 23). Fibromyalgia. Retrieved November 16, 2015, from http://emedicine.medscape.com/article/329838-overview

Tardive Dyskinesia:

Brasic, J., MD. (2015, August 12). Tardive Dyskinesia. Retrieved February 2, 2016, from http://emedicine.medscape.com/article/1151826-overview

Acute Sinusitis:

Brooke, I., MD. (2016, March 22). Acute Sinusitis. Retrieved March 28, 2016, from http://emedicine.medscape.com/article/232670-overview

Brooks, M. (n.d.). Medscape Log In. Retrieved March 13, 2016, from http://www.medscape.com/viewarticle/827493

Infective Endocarditis:

Brusch, J. (2015, October 15). Infective Endocarditis. Retrieved March 15, 2016, from http://emedicine.medscape.com/article/216650-overview

Esophageal Varices:

Buencamino, C., MD. (2015, October 1). Esophageal Varices Imaging. Retrieved March 12, 2016, from http://emedicine.medscape.com/article/367986-overview

EKG Review:

Burns, E., MD. (n.d.). LITFL ECG Library and clinical cases in cardiology. Retrieved February 8, 2016, from http://lifeinthefastlane.com/ecg-library/

Lower Gastrointestinal Bleeding:

Cagir, B., MD. (n.d.). Lower Gastrointestinal Bleeding. Retrieved March 13, 2016, from http://emedicine.medscape.com/article/188478-overview

Due Date:

Calculating a Due Date. (n.d.). Retrieved January 3, 2016, from http://www.hopkinsmedicine.org/healthlibrary/conditions/pregnancy_and_childbirth/calculating_a_due_date_85,p01209/

Cardiac Enzyme Studies:

Cardiac Enzyme Studies. (n.d.). Retrieved April 18, 2016, from http://www.webmd.com/heart-disease/cardiac-enzyme-studies

Milestones:

Carraccio, C., MD. (2015, July). *Pediatric Milestones* (Publication). https://www.acgme.org/Portals/0/PDFs/Milestones/PediatricsMilestones.pdf

Caput Succedaneum:

Case-lo, C. (2016, March 22). Caput Succedaneum (Swelling of the Scalp During Labor). Retrieved April 6, 2016, from http://www.healthline.com/health/caput-succedaneum

Upper Gastrointestinal Bleeding:

Cerulli, M., MD. (2016, March 21). Upper Gastrointestinal Bleeding. Retrieved March 26, 2016, from http://emedicine.medscape.com/article/187857-overview

Breast Cancer:

Chalasani, P., MD. (2016, February 23). Breast Cancer. Retrieved March 6, 2016, from http://emedicine.medscape.com/article/1947145-overview

Syphilis:

Chandrasekar, P. (2016, February 16). Syphilis. Retrieved February 23, 2016, from http://emedicine.medscape.com/article/229461-overview

Torsion of the Appendices:

Chang, J., MD. (2014, December 12). Torsion of the Appendices and Epididymis. Retrieved December 11, 2015, from http://emedicine.medscape.com/article/778170-overview

Measles:

Chen, S., MD. (2015, March 30). Measles. Retrieved November 15, 2015, from http://emedicine.medscape.com/article/966220-overview

Auer rods:

Chen, Y., MD. (2014, May 29). Auer rods: MedlinePlus Medical Encyclopedia Image. Retrieved November 7, 2015, from https://www.nlm.nih.gov/medlineplus/ency/imagepages/1441.htm

Down Syndrome:

Chen, H., MD. (2015, June 24). Down Syndrome. Retrieved December 4, 2015, from http://emedicine.medscape.com/article/943216-overview

Endometrial Carcinoma:

Chiang, J., MD. (2015, November 11). Premalignant Lesions of the Endometrium. Retrieved December 3, 2015, from http://emedicine.medscape.com/article/269919-overview

Chlamydia:

Chlamydia in Women/Men: Symptoms, Treatments. (n.d.). Retrieved March 14, 2016, from http://www.webmd.com/sexual-conditions/guide/chlamydia

Prostate Cancer:

Chodak, G., MD. (2015, October 15). Prostate Cancer. Retrieved April 18, 2016, from http://emedicine.medscape.com/article/1967731-overview

Glasgow Coma Scale:

Christensen, B., MD. (2014, December 5). Glasgow Coma Scale - Adult . Retrieved February 14, 2016, from http://emedicine.medscape.com/article/2172603-overview

Clark, M. A. (2012). *Pharmacology*. Philadelphia: Wolters Kluwer Health /Lippincott Williams & Wilkins.

Nephrotic Syndrome:

Cohen, E., MD. (2016, March 8). Nephrotic Syndrome. Retrieved March 21, 2016, from http://emedicine.medscape.com/article/244631-overview

Dementia With Lewy Bodies:

Crystal, H., MD. (2016, April 11). Dementia With Lewy Bodies. Retrieved April 14, 2016, from http://emedicine.medscape.com/article/1135041-overview

Bacterial Sepsis:

Cunha, B., MD. (2016, March 18). Bacterial Sepsis. Retrieved March 2, 2016, from http://emedicine.medscape.com/article/234587-overview

Pneumothorax:

Daley, B., MD. (2015, July 21). Pneumothorax. Retrieved February 06, 2016, from http://emedicine.medscape.com/article/424547-overview

Turner Syndrome:

Daniel, M., MBBS. (2015, August 7). Turner Syndrome. Retrieved November 3, 2015, from http://emedicine.medscape.com/article/949681-overview

Osteofibrous Dysplasia:

Davidson, D., MD. (2016, March 11). Osteofibrous Dysplasia. Retrieved March 23, 2016, from http://emedicine.medscape.com/article/1256595-overview

Erysipelas:

Davis, L., MD. (2015, August 11). Erysipelas. Retrieved November 21, 2015, from http://emedicine.medscape.com/article/1052445-overview

Bronchiolitis:

DeNicola, L., MD. (2015, September 1). Bronchiolitis. Retrieved December 21, 2015, from http://emedicine.medscape.com/article/961963-overview

Abruptio Placentae:

Deering, S., MD. (2015, September 14). Abruptio Placentae. Retrieved December 2, 2015, from http://emedicine.medscape.com/article/252810-overview

Croup:

Defendi, G., MD. (2015, June 17). Croup. Retrieved December 4, 2015, from http://emedicine.medscape.com/article/962972-overview

Mumps:

Defendi, G., MD. (2016, April 18). Mumps. Retrieved April 20, 2016, from http://reference.medscape.com/article/966678-overview

Antidepressants:

Depression Medications (Antidepressants). (n.d.). Retrieved January 4,

2016, from http://www.webmd.com/depression/depression-medications-antidepressants

Diseases & Conditions - Medscape Reference. (n.d.). Retrieved April 18, 2016, from http://emedicine.medscape.com/

Acute Otitis Media:

Donaldson, J., MD. (2015, February 23). Acute Otitis Media. Retrieved December 6, 2015, from http://emedicine.medscape.com/article/859316-overview

Colon Cancer:

Dragovich, T., MD. (2016, April 14). Colon Cancer. Retrieved April 18, 2016, from http://emedicine.medscape.com/article/277496-overview

Thermal Burns:

Edlich, R., MD. (2015, September 1). Thermal Burns. Retrieved February 13, 2016, from http://emedicine.medscape.com/article/1278244-overview

Lab Values:

Farinde, A., PharmD. (2014, May 14). Lab Values, Normal Adult . Retrieved November 22, 2015, from http://emedicine.medscape.com/article/2172316-overview

ACE Inhibitors:

Farinde, A., MD. (2015, August 19). ACE Inhibitors Initial Dosage Regimens . Retrieved January 15, 2016, from http://emedicine.medscape.com/article/2172124-overview

Vaccinations:

Farinde, A., PharmD. (2015, October 9). Vaccinations - Adult . Retrieved February 4, 2016, from http://emedicine.medscape.com/article/2172006-overview

Nephritis:

Fathallah-Shaykh, S., MD. (2015, October 12). Nephritis. Retrieved November 18, 2015, from

http://emedicine.medscape.com/article/982811-overview

Anal Cancer:

Fazendin, E., MD. (2016, February 9). Anal Cancer. Retrieved April 18, 2016, from http://reference.medscape.com/features/slideshow/anal-cancer

Retinal Artery Occlusion:

Feldman, B., MD. (n.d.). Retinal Artery Occlusion. Retrieved February 06, 2016, from http://emedicine.medscape.com/article/799119-overview

Pediatric Urinary Tract Infection:

Fisher, D., MD. (2015, June 18). Pediatric Urinary Tract Infection. Retrieved December 20, 2015, from http://emedicine.medscape.com/article/969643-overview

Spina Bifida:

Foster, M., MD,PhD. (2014, May 19). Spina Bifida. Retrieved November 11, 2015, from http://emedicine.medscape.com/article/311113-overview

Acute Pyelonephritis:

Fulop, T., MD. (2015, August 11). Acute Pyelonephritis. Retrieved November 3, 2015, from http://emedicine.medscape.com/article/245559-overview

Acute Pancreatitis:

Gardner, T., MD. (2015, April 1). Acute Pancreatitis. Retrieved February 11, 2016, from http://emedicine.medscape.com/article/181364-overview

Poststreptococcal Glomerulonephritis:

Geetha, D., MD. (2015, February 11). Poststreptococcal Glomerulonephritis. Retrieved December 20, 2015, from http://emedicine.medscape.com/article/240337-overview

Geitona, M. (n.d.). Medscape Log In. Retrieved February 3, 2016, from http://www.medscape.com/viewarticle/833709

Crohn Disease:

Ghazi, L., MD. (2016, February 26). Crohn Disease. Retrieved March 3, 2016, from http://emedicine.medscape.com/article/172940-overview

Phimosis and Paraphimosis:

Ghory, H., MD. (2015, September 10). Phimosis and Paraphimosis. Retrieved December 11, 2015, from http://emedicine.medscape.com/article/777539-overview

Bacterial Vaginosis:

Girerd, P., MD. (2015, November 15). Bacterial Vaginosis. Retrieved November 19, 2015, from http://emedicine.medscape.com/article/254342-overview

Epiglottitis:

Gompf, S., Dr. (n.d.). Epiglottitis. Retrieved March 13, 2016, from http://emedicine.medscape.com/article/763612-overview

Roseola Infantum:

Gorman, C., MD. (2015, October 13). Roseola Infantum. Retrieved December 11, 2015, from http://emedicine.medscape.com/article/1133023-overview

Peritonsillar Abscess:

Gosselin, B., MD. (2015, December 16). Peritonsillar Abscess. Retrieved January 17, 2016, from http://emedicine.medscape.com/article/194863-overview

Ovarian Cancer:

Green, A., MD. (2016, March 16). Ovarian Cancer. Retrieved March 24, 2016, from http://emedicine.medscape.com/article/255771-overview

Diabetic Ketoacidosis:

Hamdy, O., MD. (2015, August 13). Diabetic Ketoacidosis. Retrieved April 18, 2016, from http://emedicine.medscape.com/article/118361-overview

Legg-Calve-Perthes Disease:

Harris, G., MD. (2015, March 4). Legg-Calve-Perthes Disease. Retrieved December 23, 2015, from http://emedicine.medscape.com/article/1248267-overview

Meningitis:

Hasbun, R., MD. (2016, February 16). Meningitis. Retrieved January 19, 2016, from http://emedicine.medscape.com/article/232915-overview

Dehydration:

Haung, L., MD. (2015, December 31). Dehydration. Retrieved February 4, 2016, from http://emedicine.medscape.com/article/906999-overview

Parkinson Disease:

Hauser, R., MD. (2015, January 23). Parkinson Disease. Retrieved February 5, 2016, from http://emedicine.medscape.com/article/1831191-overview

Heart Murmurs:

Heart Murmurs Causes, Treatments, Types, and More. (n.d.). Retrieved November 17, 2015, from http://www.webmd.com/heart-disease/guide/heart-murmur-causes-treatments

Heat Rash:

Heat Rash Causes, Symptoms, Treatments, & Prevention. (n.d.). Retrieved March 12, 2016, from http://www.webmd.com/skin-problems-and-treatments/tc/heat-rash-topic-overview

Heat Stroke:

Heat Stroke: Symptoms and Treatment. (n.d.). Retrieved March 17, 2016, from http://www.webmd.com/a-to-z-guides/heat-stroke-symptoms-and-treatment

Cholelithiasis:

Heuman, D., MD. (2016, April 14). Gallstones (Cholelithiasis). Retrieved April 18, 2016, from http://emedicine.medscape.com/article/175667-overview

Candidiasis:

Hidalgo, J., MD. (2015, August 18). Candidiasis. Retrieved December 28, 2015, from http://emedicine.medscape.com/article/213853-overview

Large-Bowel Obstruction:

Hopkins, C., MD. (2015, December 9). Large-Bowel Obstruction. Retrieved February 12, 2016, from http://emedicine.medscape.com/article/774045-overview

Post-Pericardiotomy Syndrome:

Horenstein, S. M., MD. (2015, December 10). Post-Pericardiotomy Syndrome. Retrieved December 21, 2015, from http://emedicine.medscape.com/article/891471-overview

Leiomyoma:

Horner, K., MD. (2014, April 21). Leiomyoma. Retrieved November 14, 2015, from http://emedicine.medscape.com/article/1057733-overview

Surgical Knots:

E. (2011). How To Tie Surgical Knots: Instrument Tie. Retrieved April 22, 2016, from https://www.youtube.com/watch?v=-smZKFnC-U8

Surgical Knots:

E. (2011). How To Tie Surgical Knots: One-Handed Knot. Retrieved April 22, 2016, from https://www.youtube.com/watch?v=HTxT60u2Lj0

Surgical Knots:

E. (2011). How To Tie Surgical Knots: Two-Handed Knot. Retrieved April 22, 2016, from https://www.youtube.com/watch?v=_lvQ2YJ0RjQ

Cephalohematoma:

Infant Cephalohematoma. (n.d.). Retrieved February 4, 2016, from http://www.birthinjuryguide.org/birth-injury/types/cephalohematoma/

Herpes Zoster:

Janniger, C., MD. (2016, February 1). Herpes Zoster. Retrieved March 4, 2016, from http://emedicine.medscape.com/article/1132465-overview

Ischemic Stroke:

Jauch, E., MD. (2015, November 23). Ischemic Stroke. Retrieved February 4, 2016, from http://emedicine.medscape.com/article/1916852-overview

Acute Management of Stroke:

Jauch, E., MD. (2015, October 14). Acute Management of Stroke. Retrieved February 2, 2016, from http://emedicine.medscape.com/article/1159752-overview

Placenta Previa:

Joy, S., MD. (2015, March 22). Placenta Previa. Retrieved November 11, 2015, from http://emedicine.medscape.com/article/262063-overview

FAST Exam:

Juang, T., MD. (2015, September 22). Focused Assessment with Sonography in Trauma (FAST). Retrieved March 17, 2016, from http://emedicine.medscape.com/article/104363-overview

Apgar score:

Kaneshiro, N., MD. (2014, November 20). Apgar score: MedlinePlus Medical Encyclopedia. Retrieved March 1, 2016, from https://www.nlm.nih.gov/medlineplus/ency/article/003402.htm

Endometriosis:

Kapoor, D., MBBS. (2015, January 20). Endometriosis. Retrieved December 13, 2015, from http://emedicine.medscape.com/article/271899-overview

Patent Ductus Arteriosus:

Kim, L., MD. (2015, September 16). Patent Ductus Arteriosus (PDA). Retrieved January 6, 2016, from http://emedicine.medscape.com/article/891096-overview

Pressure Ulcers:

Kirman, C., MD. (2015, April 1). Pressure Ulcers and Wound Care. Retrieved February 2, 2016, from http://emedicine.medscape.com/article/190115-overview

Epilepsy and Seizures:

Ko, D., MD. (2015, November 19). Epilepsy and Seizures. Retrieved December 20, 2015, from http://emedicine.medscape.com/article/1184846-overview

Hypovolemic Shock:

Kolecki, P., MD. (2014, February 27). Hypovolemic Shock. Retrieved January 3, 2016, from http://emedicine.medscape.com/article/760145-overview

Infantile Scoliosis:

Lakshmanan, P., MBBS. (2015, November 2). Infantile Scoliosis. Retrieved December 17, 2015, from http://emedicine.medscape.com/article/1259899-overview

ACLS:

Lamberg, J., DO. (2014, March 21). ACLS - Tachycardia. Retrieved March 16, 2016, from http://emedicine.medscape.com/article/2172112-overview

Uterine Prolapse:

Lazarou, G., MD. (2016, March 27). Uterine Prolapse. Retrieved April 1, 2016, from http://emedicine.medscape.com/article/264231-overview

Hyperkalemia:

Lederer, E., MD. (2016, January 11). Hyperkalemia. Retrieved February 12, 2016, from http://emedicine.medscape.com/article/240903-overview

Hyperthyroidism:

Lee, S., MD. (2015, November 3). Hyperthyroidism. Retrieved February 11, 2016, from http://emedicine.medscape.com/article/121865-overview

Hydrocele:

Lee, S., MD. (2015, December 8). Hydrocele. Retrieved December 20, 2015, from http://emedicine.medscape.com/article/438724-overview

Polycythemia of the Newborn:

Lessaris, K., MD. (2016, January 2). Polycythemia of the Newborn. Retrieved February 3, 2016, from

http://emedicine.medscape.com/article/976319-overview

Impetigo:

Lewis, L., MD. (2016, March 31). Impetigo. Retrieved April 11, 2016, from http://emedicine.medscape.com/article/965254-overview

Glucose Tolerance Testing:

Lin, J., MBBS. (2014, March 18). Glucose Tolerance Testing. Retrieved November 13, 2015, from http://emedicine.medscape.com/article/2049402-overview

Antidotes:

List of Antidotes. (n.d.). Retrieved February 3, 2016, from http://medimoon.com/drug-information-center/list-of-antidotes/

Pediatric Headache:

Lopez, I. J., MD. (n.d.). Pediatric Headache. Retrieved March 12, 2016, from http://emedicine.medscape.com/article/2110861-overview

Reactive Arthritis:

Lozada, C., MD. (2015, October 31). Reactive Arthritis. Retrieved November 3, 2015, from http://emedicine.medscape.com/article/331347-overview

Polycystic Ovarian Syndrome:

Lucidi, R., MD. (2015, November 15). Polycystic Ovarian Syndrome. Retrieved December 3, 2015, from http://emedicine.medscape.com/article/256806-overview

Anemia:

Maakaron, J., MD. (2015, May 20). Anemia. Retrieved November 21, 2015, from http://emedicine.medscape.com/article/198475-overview

Suturing Techniques:

Mackay-Wiggan, J., MD. (2015, November 20). Suturing Techniques. Retrieved January 21, 2016, from http://emedicine.medscape.com/article/1824895-overview

Lumbosacral Radiculopathy:

Malanga, G., MD. (2015, December 30). Lumbosacral Radiculopathy. Retrieved January 18, 2016, from http://emedicine.medscape.com/article/95025-overview

Orbital Fractures:

Mathur, N., MBBS. (n.d.). Orbital Fractures. Retrieved February 13, 2016, from http://emedicine.medscape.com/article/867985-overview

De Quervain Tenosynovitis:

Meals, R., MD. (2015, August 18). De Quervain Tenosynovitis. Retrieved November 3, 2015, from http://emedicine.medscape.com/article/1243387-overview

Mallet Finger:

Meals, R., MD. (2015, August 19). Mallet Finger. Retrieved February 8, 2016, from http://emedicine.medscape.com/article/1242305-overview

Lichen Sclerosis:

Meffert, J., MD. (2016, February 24). Lichen Sclerosis et Atrophicus. Retrieved February 28, 2016, from http://emedicine.medscape.com/article/1123316-overview

Salter-Harris Fracture:

Moore, W., MD. (2015, September 5). Salter-Harris Fracture Imaging. Retrieved April 18, 2016, from http://emedicine.medscape.com/article/412956-overview

Wrist Fractures:

Morhart, M., MD. (2016, March 6). Wrist Fractures and Dislocations. Retrieved March 18, 2016, from http://emedicine.medscape.com/article/1285825-overview

Asthma:

Morris, M. (n.d.). Asthma. Retrieved March 13, 2016, from http://emedicine.medscape.com/article/296301-overview

Viral Pneumonia:

Mosenifar, Z., MD. (2015, January 13). Viral Pneumonia. Retrieved February 8, 2016, from http://emedicine.medscape.com/article/300455-overview

COPD:

Mosenifar, Z., MD. (2016, February 1). Chronic Obstructive Pulmonary Disease (COPD). Retrieved March 14, 2016, from http://emedicine.medscape.com/article/297664-overview

Geriatric Rehabilitation:

Muché, J., MD. (2016, February 25). Geriatric Rehabilitation. Retrieved March 11, 2016, from http://emedicine.medscape.com/article/318521-overview

Diabetes Management:

NDEI.org. (n.d.). Retrieved February 13, 2016, from http://www.ndei.org/AACE-guidelines-diabetes-treatment-algorithm.aspx

Transient Ischemic Attack:

Nanda, A., MD. (2015, December 1). Transient Ischemic Attack. Retrieved February 4, 2016, from http://emedicine.medscape.com/article/1910519-overview

Unconjugated Hyperbilirubinemia:

Nazer, H., MD. (2016, January 3). Unconjugated Hyperbilirubinemia. Retrieved February 5, 2016, from http://emedicine.medscape.com/article/178841-overview

Small-Bowel Obstruction:

Nobie, B., MD. (2015, January 20). Small-Bowel Obstruction. Retrieved February 4, 2016, from http://emedicine.medscape.com/article/774140-overview

Testicular Torsion:

Ogunyemi, O., MD. (2015, December 11). Testicular Torsion. Retrieved January 7, 2016, from http://emedicine.medscape.com/article/2036003-overview

Heart Failure Guidelines:

Ooi, H., MD. (2016, February 4). Heart Failure Guidelines . Retrieved March 17, 2016, from http://emedicine.medscape.com/article/2500037-overview

Primary Pulmonary Hypertension:

Oudiz, R., MD. (2016, January 27). Primary Pulmonary Hypertension. Retrieved February 5, 2016, from http://emedicine.medscape.com/article/301450-overview

Pulmonary Embolism:

Ouellette, D., MD. (n.d.). Pulmonary Embolism. Retrieved March 13, 2016, from http://emedicine.medscape.com/article/300901-overview

Acromioclavicular Joint Injury:

Owens, B., MD. (2015, August 27). Acromioclavicular Joint Injury. Retrieved November 15, 2015, from http://emedicine.medscape.com/article/92337-overview

Panesar, K., BPharmS. (n.d.). Medscape Log In. Retrieved January 11, 2016, from http://www.medscape.com/viewarticle/848348

ASD:

Pettersen, M., MD. (2016, March 2). Pediatric Complete Atrioventricular Septal Defects. Retrieved March 28, 2016, from http://emedicine.medscape.com/article/893914-overview

Phillips, D. (2015, January 17). Medscape Log In. Retrieved February 3, 2016, from http://www.medscape.com/viewarticle/838352

Colitis:

Piccoli, D., MD. (2015, September 13). Colitis. Retrieved April 18, 2016, from http://emedicine.medscape.com/article/927845-overview

Major Depression:

Preda, A., MD. (2016, October 7). Major Depression. Retrieved February 8, 2016, from http://reference.medscape.com/features/slideshow/major-depressive-disorder

Hepatitis B:

Pyrsopoulos, N., MD. (2015, January 11). Hepatitis B. Retrieved November 2, 2015, from http://emedicine.medscape.com/article/177632-overview

Skull Fracture:

Qureshi, N., MD. (2015, September 10). Skull Fracture. Retrieved February 20, 2016, from http://emedicine.medscape.com/article/248108-overview

EM Review:

REBEL Reviews - R.E.B.E.L. EM - Emergency Medicine Blog. (2014, May 10). Retrieved April 18, 2016, from http://rebelem.com/rebel-reviews/

Anticholinergic Toxicity:

Ramnarine, M., MD. (2015, August 9). Anticholinergic Toxicity. Retrieved January 7, 2016, from http://emedicine.medscape.com/article/812644-overview

Acne Vulgaris:

Rao, J., MD. (2015, December 11). Acne Vulgaris. Retrieved November 26, 2015, from http://emedicine.medscape.com/article/1069804-overview

Acute Compartment Syndrome:

Rasul, A., MD. (2015, October 20). Acute Compartment Syndrome. Retrieved January 3, 2016, from http://emedicine.medscape.com/article/307668-overview

Abdominal Hernias:

Rather, A., MD. (2015, December 1). Abdominal Hernias. Retrieved March 12, 2016, from http://emedicine.medscape.com/article/189563-overview

Heat Exhaustion:

Ratini, M., DO. (n.d.). Heat Exhaustion: Symptoms and Treatment. Retrieved March 13, 2016, from http://www.webmd.com/fitness-exercise/heat-exhaustion

Eclampsia:

Ross, M., MD. (2015, December 27). Eclampsia. Retrieved March 18, 2016, from http://emedicine.medscape.com/article/253960-overview

Gout and Pseudogout:

Rothschild, B., MD. (2016, January 31). Gout and Pseudogout. Retrieved March 4, 2016, from http://emedicine.medscape.com/article/329958-overview

Running Simple Sutures:

S. (2011). SIM SUTURE - 5. Running Simple Sutures. Retrieved April 22, 2016, from https://www.youtube.com/watch?v=ODZtJL_gb4E

Running Subcuticular Suture:

S. (2011). SIM SUTURE - 7. Running Subcuticular Suture. Retrieved April 22, 2016, from https://www.youtube.com/watch?v=iYts9c6Jrx8

Renal Cell Carcinoma:

Sachdeva, K., MD. (2015, December 8). Renal Cell Carcinoma. Retrieved February 3, 2016, from http://emedicine.medscape.com/article/281340-overview

Wernicke Encephalopathy:

Salen, P., MD. (2015, October 28). Wernicke Encephalopathy. Retrieved November 4, 2015, from http://emedicine.medscape.com/article/794583-overview

Percutaneous Abscess Drainage:

Samett, E., MD. (2014, May 2). Percutaneous Abscess Drainage. Retrieved February 21, 2016, from http://emedicine.medscape.com/article/1821039-overview

Contraception:

Samra-Latif, O., MD. (2015, August 16). Contraception. Retrieved November 20, 2015, from http://emedicine.medscape.com/article/258507-overview

Appendicitis:

Sandy, C. (n.d.). Appendicitis. Retrieved February 16, 2016, from

http://emedicine.medscape.com/article/773895-overview

Kawasaki Disease:

Scheinfeld, N., MD. (2015, September 13). Kawasaki Disease. Retrieved November 17, 2015, from http://emedicine.medscape.com/article/965367-overview

Hemolytic Anemia:

Schick, P., MD. (2015, November 15). Hemolytic Anemia. Retrieved December 2, 2015, from http://emedicine.medscape.com/article/201066-overview

Pityriasis Rosea:

Schwartz, R., MD. (2015, May 6). Pityriasis Rosea. Retrieved December 3, 2015, from http://emedicine.medscape.com/article/1107532-overview

Giant Cell Arteritis:

Seetharaman, M., MD. (n.d.). Giant Cell Arteritis (Temporal Arteritis). Retrieved March 13, 2016, from http://emedicine.medscape.com/article/332483-overview

Acute Myelogenous Leukemia:

Seiter, K., MD. (2015, November 9). Acute Myelogenous Leukemia. Retrieved December 18, 2015, from http://emedicine.medscape.com/article/197802-overview

Aortic Coarctation:

Shah, S., DO. (2014, March 27). Aortic Coarctation. Retrieved November 20, 2015, from http://emedicine.medscape.com/article/150369-overview

Anaphylaxis:

Shahzad, M. (n.d.). Anaphylaxis. Retrieved April 18, 2016, from http://emedicine.medscape.com/

Beta-Blocker:

Sharma, A., MD. (2015, January 21). Beta-Blocker Toxicity. Retrieved November 14, 2015, from

http://emedicine.medscape.com/article/813342-overview

Cystic Fibrosis:

Sharma, G., MD. (2015, July 8). Cystic Fibrosis. Retrieved November 13, 2015, from http://emedicine.medscape.com/article/1001602-overview

Thyroid Cancer:

Sharma, P., MD. (2015, February 18). Thyroid Cancer. Retrieved February 13, 2016, from http://emedicine.medscape.com/article/851968-overview

Cholangitis:

Shojamanesh, H., MD. (2015, March 11). Cholangitis. Retrieved February 2, 2016, from http://emedicine.medscape.com/article/184043-overview

Acute Conjunctivitis:

Silverman, M., MD. (2016, March 28). Acute Conjunctivitis. Retrieved April 3, 2016, from http://emedicine.medscape.com/article/797874-overview

Pediatric Pyloric Stenosis:

Singh, J., MD. (2015, July 27). Pediatric Pyloric Stenosis. Retrieved January 8, 2016, from http://emedicine.medscape.com/article/803489-overview

Trichomoniasis:

Smith, D., MD. (2015, October 21). Trichomoniasis. Retrieved December 18, 2015, from http://emedicine.medscape.com/article/230617-overview

Scarlet Fever:

Sotoodian, B., MD. (2016, March 7). Scarlet Fever. Retrieved March 18, 2016, from http://emedicine.medscape.com/article/1053253-overview

Acute Pericarditis:

Spangler, S., MD. (2014, October 6). Acute Pericarditis. Retrieved April 18, 2016, from http://emedicine.medscape.com/article/156951-overview

Kernicterus:

Springer, S., MD. (2014, April 2). Kernicterus. Retrieved January 3, 2016, from http://emedicine.medscape.com/article/975276-overview

Humerus Fracture:

Srivastava, A., MD. (2015, September 24). Humerus Fracture. Retrieved March 23, 2016, from http://emedicine.medscape.com/article/825488-overview

Acute Cholecystitis:

Steel, P., MBBS. (2015, December 27). Acute Cholecystitis and Biliary Colic. Retrieved March 1, 2016, from http://emedicine.medscape.com/article/1950020-overview

Angle Recession Glaucoma:

Sullivan, B., MD. (2015, August 17). Angle Recession Glaucoma. Retrieved November 15, 2015, from http://emedicine.medscape.com/article/1204999-overview

Unsafe medications in pregnancy:

Taking Medicine During Pregnancy: Safe and Unsafe Medications. (n.d.). Retrieved December 9, 2015, from http://www.webmd.com/baby/guide/taking-medicine-during-pregnancy

Hypertension:

The Seventh Report of the Joint National Committee on Prevention, Detection, Evaluation, and Treatment of High Blood Pressure (JNC 7). (2004). Retrieved January 4, 2016, from http://www.nhlbi.nih.gov/health-pro/guidelines/current/hypertension-jnc-7

Up and Go Test:

C. (n.d.). The Timed Up and Go Test. Retrieved January 4, 2016, from http://www.cdc.gov/steadi/pdf/tug_test-a.pdf

Endogenous Cushing Syndrome:

Thuy Nguyen, H., MD. (2015, September 3). Endogenous Cushing Syndrome. Retrieved November 13, 2015, from http://emedicine.medscape.com/article/2233083-overview

Beers Criteria:

Trucil, D. (2015, October 8). Expanded AGS Beers Criteria Offer New

Guidance, Tools For Safer Medication Use Among Older Adults Press / In The Media The American Geriatrics Society. Retrieved January 3, 2016, from http://www.americangeriatrics.org/press/id:5907

Hemorrhagic Shock:

Udeani, J., MD. (n.d.). Hemorrhagic Shock. Retrieved February 8, 2016, from http://emedicine.medscape.com/article/432650-overview

Genital Herpes:

Ural, S., MD. (2015, April 16). Genital Herpes in Pregnancy. Retrieved December 21, 2015, from http://emedicine.medscape.com/article/274874-overview

Urinary Incontinence:

Vasavada, S., MD. (2015, October 27). Urinary Incontinence. Retrieved February 7, 2016, from http://emedicine.medscape.com/article/452289-overview

Otitis Externa:

Waitzman, A., MD. (2015, August 13). Otitis Externa. Retrieved December 18, 2015, from http://emedicine.medscape.com/article/994550-overview

Waszynski, C., RN. (n.d.). Medscape Log In. Retrieved February 5, 2016, from http://www.medscape.com/viewarticle/481726

ADHD:

Wilkes, M., MD. (2016, April 4). Pediatric Attention Deficit Hyperactivity Disorder (ADHD). Retrieved April 7, 2016, from http://emedicine.medscape.com/article/912633-overview

Cirrhosis:

Wolf, D., MD. (2015, December 3). Cirrhosis. Retrieved December 21, 2015, from http://emedicine.medscape.com/article/185856-overview

Nephrolithiasis:

Wolf, S. J., MD. (2015, October 30). Nephrolithiasis. Retrieved March 12, 2016, from http://emedicine.medscape.com/article/437096-overview

Nursemaid Elbow:

Wolfram, W., MD. (2016, February 7). Nursemaid Elbow. Retrieved February 28, 2016, from http://emedicine.medscape.com/article/803026-overview

Gonorrhea:

Wong, B., MD. (2016, March 15). Gonorrhea. Retrieved March 18, 2016, from http://emedicine.medscape.com/article/218059-overview

Cardiac Tamponade:

Yarlagadda, C., MD. (2015, January 27). Cardiac Tamponade. Retrieved November 6, 2015, from http://emedicine.medscape.com/article/152083-overview

Erythema Infectiosum:

Zellman, G., MD. (2015, November 17). Erythema Infectiosum. Retrieved December 6, 2015, from http://emedicine.medscape.com/article/1132078-overview

Alteplase:

Alteplase (Rx)Brand and Other Names:Activase, TPA, more...Cathflo Activase. (n.d.). Retrieved March 3, 2016, from http://reference.medscape.com/drug/activase-tpa-alteplase-342287

HPV Vaccine:

Human papillomavirus vaccine, quadrivalent (Rx)Brand and Other Names:Gardasil, hpv vaccine, quadrivalent. (n.d.). Retrieved January 3, 2016, from http://reference.medscape.com/drug/gardasil-human-papillomavirus-vaccine-quadrivalent-343111

Aortic Dissection:

Mancini, M., MD. (2015, December 2). Aortic Dissection. Retrieved February 14, 2016, from http://emedicine.medscape.com/article/2062452-overview

Prothrombin:

Prothrombin complex concentrate, human (Rx)Brand and Other Names:Kcentra. (n.d.). Retrieved February 13, 2016, from http://reference.medscape.com/drug/kcentra-prothrombin-complex-concentrate-human-999848

Hemorrhoids:

Thornton, S., MD. (2015, December 29). Hemorrhoids. Retrieved February 1, 2016, from http://emedicine.medscape.com/article/775407-overview

APA formatting by BibMe.org.

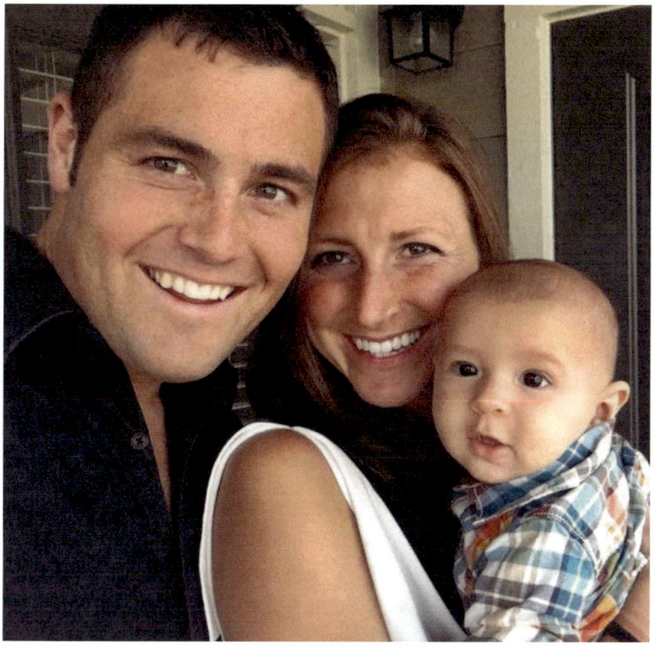

Aaron Shaw is a transplanted Ohioan who is living and practicing as a Neurosurgical Physician Assistant in central Texas. Aaron grew up in Ohio and delivered newspapers for 13 years and worked as a nursing aide during elementary and high school before heading Bowling Green State University for his BS in Applied Health Science. He married his best friend, Valerie VanRavenswaay from Ontario, Canada his freshmen year at 19 years old, after they met at a Christian convention in Dunville, ON. Valerie and Aaron have lived the last decade investing in their medical education so that they can positively impact patients' lives directly. After earning his undergraduate degree, Aaron later obtained two Masters Degrees in Exercise Physiology and Biomedical Science (Physician Assistant) at the University of Toledo Medical Center. His wife is currently a medical resident/ physician, in College Station Texas, after completing her degree in Osteopathic Medicine from the Ohio University Heritage College of Osteopathic Medicine. They now have a baby boy, Jakx, and are adjusting to their medical careers and new life as a family.

Made in the USA
Las Vegas, NV
03 November 2026

57422977R00145